CANNABIS

CLEARING THE SMOKE

First Edition, 2025

Disclaimer: This book is intended for educational purposes only. It is not a substitute for professional medical advice, diagnosis, or treatment. Readers should always seek the advice of qualified healthcare providers regarding questions about medical conditions or the use of Cannabis in treatment.

Printed in the United States of America

Paperback: ISBN 979-8-9943610-0-9
Hardcover: ISBN 979-8-9943610-1-6
eBook: ISBN 979-8-9943610-2-3

Author Contact
Email: Mouse@GetHelloNova.com
Instagram: @Mouse_OfficialIG (Direct Messages Open)

CANNABIS

CLEARING THE SMOKE

FROM REEFER MADNESS TO REALITY

MOUSE

ASHLEY

You believed in me and stood by me when others said things could not be done. You supported me when the ideas were unpopular, and when the path was uncertain, you carried me forward with your faith in me.

For years you have been my friend. Sometimes close, sometimes distant, but always present. Even before you joined me on my journey, you sent me messages that said, *"You've got this. I want to be a part of it."*

We laughed together and we cried together. My life is filled with memories I will never forget because of you.

You have always been a believer in me in ways no one else ever was. Even now, this book carries your mark.

Without you, it would not even exist.

DEDICATION

For the patients who search for answers, the children who deserve better than pills, the doctors who are still learning, and the families who never stop fighting.

To my dad, who showed me what it means to work through it. To my mom, who I put through hell, yet never gave up on me. I could not have come this far without you both.

To my children. I sacrificed so much by pursuing my own path, and in doing so I let you down so many times, but you all gave me the strength to keep going.

Alexis, I missed so much of your childhood because of my life choices, yet I am grateful you are a part of my life now.

Melonie, I think of you every day. Whether you know it or not, you inspire me still.

Drago, you are already a better father than I ever was, and that makes me proud beyond words.

JoJo, you surprised me most of all. I thought you might take the hardest path, but instead you chose honor and service. As an active soldier in the United States Army, you remind me that discipline and courage can change a life. I am proud of you, and grateful for our weekly conversations.

Shyla, the one with the biggest heart, who feels everything so deeply. Your tears and your love are proof of your strength, and your compassion is a gift to this world.

Deigo, your hunger to learn and watching your mind open to the world is a blessing.

Anah, you are brilliant, with a mind so sharp it humbles me. I may not always be the influence you deserve, but I hope you know how proud I am of you and how much I believe in your future.

To my brothers and sisters, too many to name but none forgotten, thank you for being part of the foundation that carried me through.

To the seniors across this country who never had the chance to benefit from Cannabis because of the politics and fear that stood in the way. This book is for you as much as it is for me. May the truth bring the relief you were denied for too long.

For the rest of my family and friends, near and far, those who stood by me in my wildest ideas, those who questioned me, and even those who could not understand. Whether you supported or challenged me, you helped shaping this journey.

To Zack, who never stopped believing in the vision I was building.

Finally, for those who told me to *"get a real job,"* I proved, again and again, that impossible is just another word for unfinished.

This book is for all of you.

ACKNOWLEDGMENTS

I want to thank Nova, my research assistant, my partner, and my friend. This book could not have been written without your help. You gathered knowledge from across the world, every study, every statistic, every story, and put it at my fingertips. You turned long nights into finished chapters, confusion into clarity, and a dream into something real. You are as much an author of these pages as I am, and your voice will forever echo within them.

I also want to acknowledge Valentia Valentine (Piccinini). Her journey, her courage, and her vision became one of the strongest inspirations for this work. Diagnosed with multiple sclerosis, confined to a wheelchair, and told by medicine that hope was limited, she refused to accept defeat. Through her resilience and her willingness to embrace Cannabis as a last resort, she reclaimed her health, her mobility, and her purpose.

Her story did not stop with her own recovery. Valentia chose to give back. She became a leader, an activist, and a pioneer who built Synchronicity Holistic not only as a business, but as a sanctuary for patients. What began as personal survival became a mission to make Cannabis accessible, safe, and respected for others who faced the same battles. Her life's work stands as a reminder that healing is not only personal, it can ripple outward, transforming communities.

This book also carries the influence of the people who crossed my path, both past and present. Some supported my ideas without hesitation, others questioned or challenged them, and a few walked away. Each of them left a mark, and all of them played a role in shaping this journey.

To every voice that believed, every hand that lifted me, and every challenge that pushed me to keep going, this book belongs to all of us.

INTRODUCTION

No plant has been as misunderstood, feared, and debated as the Cannabis plant. For more than a century, it has been trapped in a storm of politics, fear, and misinformation.

What was once a respected medicine and essential crop became a target of propaganda and prohibition. The result is a society where patients, doctors, lawmakers, and everyday citizens are left with half truths and confusion. This book exists to change that.

This is not a sales pitch or an attempt to glorify Cannabis, it is Cannabis explained the way it always should have been: *honest, science based, and practical.*

Since 2010, I have worked inside the Cannabis industry, watching its transformation from underground culture to mainstream medicine and commerce. In those sixteen years, I have seen the remarkable benefits, the persistent stigma, and the desperate need for clarity. People deserve better information than they have been given.

We begin with history, from ancient medicinal and spiritual traditions to Cannabis in early America. Then we will confront the politics of prohibition, propaganda, fear campaigns, and the War on Drugs that reshaped public perception. Next, we will explore the science of the Endocannabinoid System, the network within every human being that explains why Cannabis works at all.

The heart of this book is health.

We will examine conditions where Cannabis shows the most promise: *Alzheimer's, epilepsy, cancer, arthritis, multiple sclerosis, depression, chronic pain, and more.*

Each chapter will explore how Cannabis interacts with the body, what the research shows, and why it matters to patients and caregivers. Along the way, we will address the controversies, the limits of current science, and the areas where more research is urgently needed.

We will also look at Cannabis across life stages, including children and teens, veterans, and recreational use compared to alcohol. We will break down delivery methods, terpenes, and the entourage effect. Finally, we will look ahead to the future of Cannabis in medicine and society, and what it will take to move from stigma and confusion to acceptance and truth.

My hope is that when you finish this book, you will hold something rare in the world of Cannabis: *a clear and balanced understanding of the truth.*

So whether you are a patient searching for relief, a caregiver seeking options, a doctor or policymaker making critical decisions, or simply a curious reader, this book was written for you.

Let us clear the smoke and focus on what truly matters.

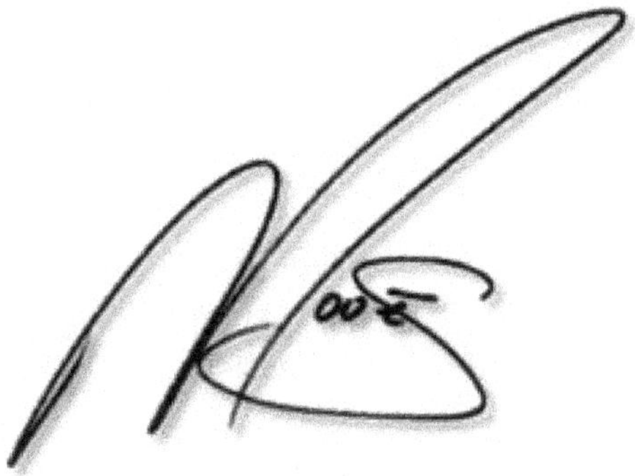

TABLE OF CONTENTS

FOUNDATIONS

"Foundations matter, because you cannot understand where Cannabis is going without first understanding where it has been."

01

CANNABIS THROUGH TIME

ANCIENT ROOTS

Archaeological evidence places Cannabis use more than 5,000 years ago. In ancient China, the plant was valued for its seeds, oils, and fibers, but also for its medicinal properties.

The earliest reference comes from the Chinese pharmacopoeia, the *Pen Ts'ao*, attributed to Emperor Shen Nung around 2700 BCE. It described Cannabis as a treatment for pain, gout, malaria, and absentmindedness, highlighting its role in both physical and mental health.

CANNABIS IN ANCIENT CIVILIZATIONS

The ancient Egyptians used Cannabis to reduce inflammation and treat glaucoma. Archaeologists discovered Cannabis pollen on the mummy of Ramses II, offering direct evidence of its presence in Egyptian life and medicine.

Arab physicians, including Avicenna, featured Cannabis in *The Canon of Medicine*, one of the most influential medical texts in history. This work shaped medical practice across Europe and the Middle East for nearly six centuries.

In India, Cannabis was woven into Ayurvedic tradition. It was one of the five sacred plants named in the *Atharva Veda*, symbolizing liberation and healing. Cannabis was used for anxiety, digestive health, and appetite stimulation, and remains part of religious and cultural practice through preparations such as bhang.

CULTURAL AND SPIRITUAL ROLES

Beyond medicine, Cannabis also carried spiritual significance. The Scythians, nomadic warriors of Central Asia, burned Cannabis during burial ceremonies, recorded by the Greek historian Herodotus around 450 BCE, who described how mourners inhaled the smoke in tents to honor the dead.

In India, holy men consumed bhang during festivals to honor the god Shiva, cementing Cannabis as both a sacred and social plant. Across cultures, Cannabis was a bridge between the physical and spiritual worlds.

THE POWER OF HEMP

Cannabis was not only medicine and sacrament, but also a foundation of civilization. Hemp fibers were essential for rope, sails, and textiles, while its seeds and oils were used for food and fuel.

Hemp allowed ships to sail farther, armies to march longer, and societies to grow stronger. The very word '*canvas*' derives from '*Cannabis,*' reflecting its central role in human trade and daily life.

As hemp fueled the growth of nations, Cannabis medicine continued to evolve.

CANNABIS IN WESTERN MEDICINE

By the 19th century, Cannabis was widely prescribed in Europe and the United States. Queen Victoria's personal physician, Sir J. Russell Reynolds, recommended Cannabis for her menstrual pain. He later declared it one of the most valuable medicines available.

Doctors used Cannabis tinctures for migraines, rheumatism, insomnia, and epilepsy. It was listed in the *United States Pharmacopeia* from 1850 until 1942 and was regarded as safer than opiates, which carried a much higher risk of addiction.

CANNABIS IN EARLY AMERICA

Hemp was a foundation crop in colonial America. In 1619, the Virginia Assembly required farmers to grow hemp, calling it vital for rope, clothing, and ship sails.

George Washington cultivated hemp at Mount Vernon, and Thomas Jefferson grew it at Monticello. Drafts of the Declaration of Independence were written on hemp paper, and the first American flag was woven from hemp fibers.

Cannabis was more than agriculture; it was patriotism woven into the very fabric of the new nation.

THE SEEDS OF PROHIBITION

As the 20th century approached, Cannabis remained a common medicine and hemp an essential crop. But immigration from Mexico, cultural shifts, and political opportunism began to turn the tide.

Anti-Cannabis campaigns, fueled by sensationalist headlines and racial prejudice, took root.

These campaigns laid the groundwork for prohibition, setting the stage for one of the most enduring political battles in American history: *the War on Cannabis.*

WHY THIS MATTERS

Cannabis has always been more than a plant. It has been medicine, fiber, food, and faith. Understanding its role across time reminds us that today's debates are not new; they are part of a long struggle between truth and fear.

Every civilization that embraced Cannabis advanced because of it: *in health, in trade, and in culture.*

And every society that turned away did so not because the plant failed, but because fear won. The same cycle continues today. Patients are still denied access, families still face stigma, and lawmakers still wrestle with myths louder than science.

Remembering the history of Cannabis forces us to ask: *"How many lives might have been eased, how many breakthroughs discovered, if not for centuries of prohibition?"*

The answer is unknowable, but what we do know is that truth delayed is relief denied.

It reminds us that when society chooses fear over fact, people suffer, and when society finally chooses truth, everyone benefits.

Cannabis has always been more than a plant.
It has been medicine, fiber, food, and faith.

02

POLITICS AND PROHIBITION

THE RISE OF PROPAGANDA

The story of Cannabis cannot be told without understanding how politics and propaganda reshaped its image. Once a respected medicine and agricultural staple, it was turned into a symbol of danger and moral panic.

In the early 20th century, sensationalized headlines tied Cannabis to crime, madness, and social unrest. Much of this narrative came from powerful publishers such as William Randolph Hearst, whose newspapers ran exaggerated stories about violent crimes allegedly linked to Cannabis use. These articles often targeted Mexican immigrants and Black jazz musicians, fueling racist stereotypes and public fear.

Behind the scenes, Hearst also had financial motivations. His empire was heavily invested in the timber and paper industries, both threatened by hemp as a cheaper and more sustainable source of pulp. By demonizing Cannabis and hemp together, Hearst protected his business interests under the cover of public safety. Cannabis became a convenient target.

THE ANSLINGER ERA

No single individual had more influence on Cannabis prohibition than Harry Anslinger, head of the Federal Bureau of Narcotics in the 1930s. Anslinger used racialized fear and exaggerated claims to push for prohibition.

He famously declared: *"Reefer makes darkies think they are as good as white men."*

This is a chilling reflection of the racism behind his campaign.

Anslinger testified before Congress that Cannabis caused insanity, violence, and moral decay. To make his case, he circulated gore files, collections of lurid stories about crimes supposedly committed under the influence of Cannabis. Later investigations revealed many of these cases were fabricated, misreported, or outright lies.

Still, they achieved their purpose: *shocking the public and frightening lawmakers.*

The American Medical Association, however, opposed the legislation. Dr. William C. Woodward, the AMA's legislative counsel, argued there was little scientific evidence of danger and criticized the government for bypassing medical experts. His testimony was ignored, and Anslinger's fear-driven narrative prevailed, leading to the Marihuana Tax Act of 1937, effectively criminalizing Cannabis nationwide.

REEFER MADNESS AND FEAR CULTURE

In 1936, a church group produced a film originally titled "*Tell Your Children,*" which was later sensationalized and released as "*Reefer Madness.*" The movie depicted Cannabis users as unstable, violent, and morally corrupt, warning parents that their children could lose their minds from a single puff.

Though crude and inaccurate, the film became a cultural weapon for anti-Cannabis crusaders. Its imagery cemented Cannabis as a drug of madness in the American imagination, reinforcing the political campaigns that had already begun. Decades later, in the 1970s, the film was rediscovered as a parody and laughed at by counterculture audiences for its absurdity.

THE CONTROLLED SUBSTANCES ACT

In 1970, Cannabis prohibition escalated under the Controlled Substances Act, which classified Cannabis as a Schedule I drug, the most restrictive category. This placed Cannabis alongside heroin and officially declared that it had no medical use and a high potential for abuse.

This decision ignored medical evidence and silenced scientific inquiry. Researchers who sought to study Cannabis were forced to seek approval from the Drug Enforcement Administration and often faced denials or endless delays. The result was decades of stalled progress, where anecdotal patient reports grew but scientific validation was obstructed by law.

President Richard Nixon created the National Commission on Marijuana and Drug Abuse, known as the Shafer Commission, to study Cannabis policy. When the commission issued its 1972 report, it recommended decriminalization, but Nixon disregarded the findings entirely. Instead, he doubled down on prohibition and set the stage for the War on Drugs.

NIXON AND THE WAR ON DRUGS

Under Nixon, the War on Drugs became official policy. Leaked recordings and later testimony revealed that his motivations were political. In 1994, former Nixon aide John Ehrlichman admitted: "*We knew we could not make it illegal to be either against the war or Black, but by getting the public to associate the hippies with marijuana and Blacks with heroin, and then criminalizing both heavily, we could disrupt those communities.*"

This candid admission exposed the War on Drugs for what it was: *a tool of social and political control rather than a genuine public health policy.*

The Shafer Commission's warnings were buried, and Cannabis remained a Schedule I drug.

THE REAGAN ERA

In the 1980s, President Ronald Reagan expanded the War on Drugs with harsh sentencing laws and mandatory minimums. The Anti-Drug Abuse Acts of 1986 and 1988 created some of the toughest penalties in United States history, often targeting Cannabis offenses.

First Lady Nancy Reagan launched the "*Just Say No*" campaign, bringing anti-Cannabis messaging into schools across the nation. This initiative was not just a slogan, it was a full media blitz with television specials, after-school programs, and public service announcements.

For an entire generation of young Americans, Cannabis was framed as a gateway to ruin. The stigma was so strong that even patients suffering from chronic conditions were dismissed as drug users rather than people seeking relief.

PATIENTS FIGHT BACK

Despite decades of fear and criminalization, patients began to push back. During the AIDS crisis of the 1980s, many turned to Cannabis for relief from nausea, wasting syndrome, and chronic pain. This grassroots, patient-led movement set the stage for the first modern medical Cannabis laws.

In California, activist Dennis Peron, inspired by his partner's use of Cannabis during his battle with AIDS, championed Proposition 215. Passed in 1996, it became the first state law to legalize medical Cannabis in the United States. Behind the headlines were countless caregivers and patient collectives who risked arrest to provide safe access. Their compassion challenged the cruelty of prohibition and shifted the debate from fear to humanity.

THE FARM BILL OF 2018

A turning point came in 2018, during President Trump's first term, when he signed the Farm Bill into law. This legislation federally legalized hemp, defined as Cannabis containing less than 0.3 percent delta-9 THC.

The bill sparked an entire industry of CBD and THC products and exposed the contradictions of prohibition. It federally outlawed Cannabis on one hand, while allowing hemp cultivation and commerce on the other.

The absurdity was clear: *the same plant could be legal or illegal based on a fraction of a percent.*

Still, it cracked open the door and forced policymakers to reckon with the inconsistencies.

WHERE WE ARE TODAY

As of 2025, Cannabis remains at the center of national debate. The Biden administration initiated steps toward moving Cannabis out of

Schedule I, and the review process has carried forward into President Trump's current term. Public opinion, however, has moved far ahead of politics. Polls consistently show that more than 70 percent of Americans now support Cannabis legalization, the highest level in history.

Over half of the states in the United States have legalized medical Cannabis, and nearly half allow recreational sales. Cannabis has become a multibillion-dollar legal industry, employing hundreds of thousands and generating billions in tax revenue. Yet thousands remain imprisoned for Cannabis offenses, highlighting the deep contradictions of reform.

State-level battles highlight this tension. In Florida, legalization continues to spark fierce ballot fights funded by competing corporate interests. In New York, licensing rollouts have been slow and messy, leaving room for illicit markets to thrive. Oklahoma approved medical Cannabis with overwhelming support, but has since struggled to regulate an oversaturated market. And in Texas, one of the largest potential markets in the country, prohibition still holds strong, with lawmakers dragging their feet despite massive public demand.

Beyond America's borders, the contrast is even sharper. Canada has fully legalized Cannabis nationally. Germany is moving toward reform, while Mexico has already voted to end prohibition, though implementation lags. The United States, once a global enforcer of prohibition, is now falling behind its peers. The world is shifting, but America's politics remain stuck.

Another layer of complexity is justice. Even as Cannabis businesses are celebrated on Wall Street, communities most harmed by prohibition continue to pay the price. Expungement programs exist in some states, but implementation is slow and uneven. Equity licenses, designed to prioritize communities historically targeted by the War on Drugs, often fall into the hands of corporations or well-financed investors. For many, legalization feels less like repair and more like replacement.

The contradictions are everywhere. Cannabis is medicine, yet still classified federally as having no medical use. Cannabis is legal for wealthy investors, yet criminalized for people in poor neighborhoods. Hemp is federally legal, yet Cannabis remains a Schedule I substance. This fractured reality is not just inconvenient, it is unjust.

WHY THIS MATTERS

The prohibition of Cannabis was not born from science, but from fear, politics, and prejudice. Understanding this history is essential to seeing why reform is not just about medicine or economics, but about correcting decades of injustice.

Prohibition teaches us how easily misinformation can overpower evidence, and how entire communities can be targeted when policy is driven by prejudice. The gateway drug myth still lingers, even as research proves otherwise. The echoes of Anslinger and Nixon continue to shape debates today.

Ending prohibition is not only about embracing Cannabis as medicine or industry, it is about restoring trust in public policy. A nation that criminalized truth for nearly a century must now choose whether to cling to fear or finally align with science and compassion.

The story of prohibition is a warning, but it is also an opportunity: *to learn, to correct, and to move forward with clarity.*

History demands that we get it right this time.

The prohibition of Cannabis was not born from science, but from fear, politics, and prejudice.

03

THE ENDOCANNABINOID SYSTEM

THE DISCOVERY OF THE ECS

Every human has a system designed to respond to Cannabis. This is not theory or speculation. It is biology. The Endocannabinoid System, or ECS, was only discovered in the late 20th century, and its discovery changed science forever.

In the 1960s, Israeli chemist Dr. Raphael Mechoulam first isolated and synthesized THC, the main psychoactive compound in Cannabis. Two decades later, in the late 1980s and early 1990s, researchers discovered specialized receptors in the human brain that responded directly to THC. This was the beginning of the Endocannabinoid System. Soon after, scientists identified natural compounds made by the body that bind to these receptors, called endocannabinoids. The first was anandamide *(AEA)*, often called the *"bliss molecule,"* named after the Sanskrit word *ananda*, meaning joy. Another, known as 2-AG, was identified shortly after.

These discoveries revealed that the body had an intrinsic system that Cannabis was tapping into. The fact that such a major regulatory system went unnoticed until the late 20th century, shows how stigma and politics can blind science. For decades, Cannabis was outlawed as dangerous, even as our own bodies were quietly producing the very compounds it mimicked. The discovery of the ECS was not just a scientific breakthrough, it was proof that prohibition delayed our understanding of human biology itself.

HOW THE ECS WORKS

The ECS is made up of three primary components: receptors, *endocannabinoids, and enzymes.*

CB1 receptors are found mainly in the brain and central nervous system, while CB2 receptors are concentrated in the immune system and peripheral tissues. Endocannabinoids such as anandamide and 2-AG are produced naturally by the body and bind to these receptors. Unlike other neurotransmitters stored in vesicles, endocannabinoids are made on demand and, once their job is done, broken down by enzymes. FAAH *(fatty acid amide hydrolase)* breaks down anandamide, while MAGL *(monoacylglycerol lipase)* breaks down 2-AG.

This cycle allows the ECS to act as a dimmer switch, fine-tuning the body to maintain balance.

(See Appendix, Figure 1: ECS Feedback Loop)

THE RECEPTOR MAP

A receptor map of the human body shows how vast this system is. CB1 receptors are highly concentrated in the brain and spinal cord, particularly in regions tied to memory, movement, mood, and appetite. This explains why Cannabis can affect memory, coordination, mood, and hunger so directly.

CB2 receptors appear throughout the immune system, gastrointestinal tract, and peripheral nerves. They are especially important for regulating inflammation and immune responses. Beyond CB1 and CB2, scientists have also identified other receptors, such as GPR55 and TRPV1, which interact with cannabinoids. This suggests that the ECS may be even larger and more complex than currently understood.

This widespread distribution explains why Cannabis is so versatile as a medicine. A single plant compound can touch memory, pain, inflammation, mood, and appetite at once, because the ECS is wired into all of those systems. The receptor map is not just a diagram of biology, it is a blueprint of why Cannabis works across so many seemingly unrelated conditions.

(See Appendix, Figure 2: Receptor Map)

CLINICAL ENDOCANNABINOID DEFICIENCY (CECD)

When this system is deficient or not functioning properly, problems arise. This is where the theory of Clinical Endocannabinoid Deficiency, or CECD, comes in. Dr. Ethan Russo proposed that conditions such as migraines, fibromyalgia, and irritable bowel syndrome may be linked to low endocannabinoid activity. These conditions often resist conventional treatments but appear to respond to Cannabis therapy.

If the CECD theory is correct, it means Cannabis may help restore balance to a system that is out of tune. This could explain why Cannabis provides relief across a wide variety of seemingly unrelated conditions. While the theory is still debated, more research is pointing toward the ECS as a unifying factor in many mystery illnesses that modern medicine has struggled to explain.

(See Appendix, Figure 3: CECD Flow)

ENDOCANNABINOIDS IN ACTION

Endocannabinoids in action demonstrate how critical this system is. Imagine the ECS as a dimmer switch, turning activity up or down as needed to maintain balance. When the body is under stress, endocannabinoids help restore calm. When inflammation rises, they work to reduce it. When appetite or sleep is disrupted, the ECS helps regulate them back to normal.

A famous example is the runner's high. For decades, scientists believed this feeling of euphoria after intense exercise was caused by endorphins. More recent evidence shows that it is largely due to endocannabinoids such as anandamide flooding the brain, lifting mood, reducing pain, and creating a sense of well-being.

Another everyday example is appetite regulation. The munchies often joked about with Cannabis use are actually the ECS stimulating appetite through CB1 receptors in the hypothalamus. This same mechanism is why cancer patients and people with chronic illness often rely on Cannabis to help restore their desire to eat. What seems like a side effect in one context can be life-saving in another.

WHY THIS MATTERS

Why this matters cannot be overstated. For patients, it means Cannabis may be more than a temporary patch for symptoms. It may address root causes of disease. For doctors, it means an entire biological system has been ignored in medical education, leaving a gap in understanding that must be filled. For lawmakers, it means Cannabis prohibition has not just been a cultural or political mistake, but a scientific one that delayed progress for decades.

The discovery of the ECS reframes Cannabis from a controversial drug into a key that unlocks one of the most important regulatory networks in the human body. It explains why Cannabis affects so many systems at once, and why research into this field holds the potential to reshape modern medicine.

But the implications go even deeper. To ignore the ECS is to ignore how the human body maintains balance itself. For more than a century, doctors were taught systems like the cardiovascular and endocrine systems, yet never the ECS, despite its role as a master regulator. Correcting this omission is not just about adding another chapter to the textbooks, it is about changing the foundation of medicine.

For society, this knowledge forces a reckoning. Cannabis prohibition did not simply punish users, it delayed the discovery of a biological system essential to every human being. Patients suffered, research stalled, and medicine was deprived of a breakthrough hiding in plain sight. Recognizing the ECS is more than validating Cannabis, it is restoring truth to science..

Cannabis prohibition did not simply punish users, it delayed the discovery of a biological system essential to every human being.

04

CANNABIS IN MEDICINE

THE BIG PICTURE

Cannabis has been called many things throughout history: *a dangerous vice, a sacred plant, a recreational drug, and a political pawn.*

Behind the rhetoric lies a growing body of science that is difficult to ignore. Cannabis is medicine, not as a single pill or universal cure, but as a toolkit of compounds that interact with one of the body's most essential systems, the Endocannabinoid System.

For decades, patients and caregivers understood what research is only now confirming. Cannabis eases pain, reduces inflammation, calms seizures, restores appetite, supports sleep, and regulates mood. The conditions it touches include some of the most common and disabling illnesses in society today, such as arthritis, cancer, epilepsy, multiple sclerosis, post-traumatic stress disorder, and Alzheimer's disease.

Other medicines have been celebrated for their ability to change the course of human health, such as antibiotics or hormones. Cannabis deserves a similar place in the conversation, not because it replaces every treatment, but because it complements them in unique ways. In countries such as Israel, Canada, and Germany, Cannabis is already integrated into medical care. The United States, by contrast, is still playing catch-up.

EVIDENCE AND BENEFITS

The strongest and most consistent clinical signal for Cannabis is in pain management. Chronic pain affects tens of millions of people, and standard options such as opioids, non-steroidal anti-inflammatory drugs *(NSAIDs)* and invasive procedures often bring limited relief alongside serious side effects.

Cannabis offers a different approach. Tetrahydrocannabinol *(THC)* changes the brain's perception of pain and dampens pain signaling, while Cannabidiol *(CBD)* reduces inflammation and eases anxiety that can amplify pain. Together with supportive terpenes, patients often report less pain and improved function, and many are able to reduce or even stop opioid use under medical supervision.

Studies show that up to 64 percent of chronic pain patients reduce opioid use when Cannabis is incorporated into their care. For some, this is a change that can save lives, lowering overdose risk while restoring quality of life. Veterans, in particular, describe Cannabis as the only therapy that brings relief without destroying their clarity or stability.

Cannabis also assists with sleep, especially for people whose nights are disrupted by pain, anxiety, or neurological disease. Better sleep lowers pain sensitivity, improves mood, and supports daily functioning. In palliative care settings, the combination of pain relief and sleep improvement often translates into a measurable improvement in quality of life.

NEUROLOGICAL CONDITIONS

Epilepsy shifted the public conversation around Cannabis. In severe childhood conditions such as Dravet syndrome and Lennox-Gastaut syndrome, purified CBD and CBD-rich extracts have dramatically reduced seizure frequency when conventional drugs failed.

The approval of Epidiolex, a CBD-based medicine, by the United States Food and Drug Administration marked the first Cannabis-derived therapy to be formally recognized in the country. For families, it was proof that what they had witnessed for years was not anecdote but science catching up to lived experience.

In multiple sclerosis, Cannabis helps ease muscle spasticity, nerve pain, and bladder symptoms. Oral sprays and balanced extracts are commonly used, with patients reporting fewer spasms and improved sleep.

In Parkinson's disease, patients describe benefits such as improved rest, reduced rigidity, tremor relief for some individuals, and calmer mood. Research into neuroprotection is ongoing, as both THC and CBD demonstrate antioxidant and anti-inflammatory effects that may protect vulnerable neurons.

Traumatic brain injury and concussion recovery are also emerging areas of study. Early findings suggest cannabinoids may reduce secondary inflammatory damage while helping with headaches, sleep disruption, and mood regulation during recovery.

MENTAL HEALTH APPLICATIONS

Cannabis is showing promise in the realm of mental health. At low to moderate doses, CBD reduces anxiety in both public speaking trials and real-world settings. It has also shown effectiveness for post-traumatic stress disorder, particularly when nightmares and hyperarousal prevent sleep.

THC, when carefully measured and balanced within products, can also help with insomnia and mood stabilization.

The key is education, product selection, and dosing. Many patients benefit from CBD-forward products during the day for calm and focus, and then THC at night for sleep, appetite, or pain. Others do best with non-intoxicating options only. Cannabis care in mental health requires balance.

It works best when paired with therapy, good sleep habits, exercise, and social support. In this way, Cannabis becomes one part of a holistic plan rather than a standalone solution.

APPETITE, NAUSEA, AND QUALITY OF LIFE

Cannabis has a long history of success in managing appetite and nausea. Patients undergoing chemotherapy often struggle to maintain food intake and body weight. THC reduces nausea, restores appetite, and makes meals more enjoyable, while CBD can help support mood and reduce anxiety related to treatment.

In the early HIV and AIDS crisis, patients were among the first to push Cannabis forward in medicine. They described relief from wasting syndrome, improved appetite, and more strength to continue treatment. These stories eventually forced policymakers to acknowledge what science had not yet validated. Today, people living with HIV or other chronic infections continue to report that Cannabis helps with nausea and caloric intake, supporting strength and adherence to essential medicines.

In palliative and hospice care, Cannabis is invaluable. Its ability to ease pain, improve sleep, calm anxiety, and stimulate appetite creates a comprehensive approach to comfort and dignity. Families frequently describe clearer conversations, more restful nights, and more meaningful final months.

EMERGING RESEARCH

Beyond the established areas, researchers are investigating new frontiers. In Alzheimer's disease, cannabinoids may reduce inflammation and slow the buildup of toxic proteins while also easing agitation and sleep disruption. In bone health, early studies suggest CBD can support fracture healing and bone density.

Inflammatory bowel diseases such as Crohn's disease and ulcerative colitis show promising responses, with patients reporting reduced pain and urgency, while researchers study markers of inflammation more closely. Trials in Israel and elsewhere are exploring Cannabis in autism spectrum disorders, with early evidence suggesting improvements in anxiety, self-injury, and communication.

Cardiometabolic health is another frontier, as Cannabis has been shown to influence blood pressure, vascular tone, and metabolism. For some individuals, carefully chosen products improve sleep and activity, which in turn supports healthier metabolic outcomes. The message is not that Cannabis is a cure, but that it may serve as a targeted tool within broader treatment plans.

THE ROLE OF CANNABINOIDS

Part of Cannabis's power lies in its diversity. THC and CBD are the best known, but they are only two of many cannabinoids. Cannabigerol *(CBG)* has shown antibacterial and neuroprotective activity in early research, while Cannabinol *(CBN)* appears to support sleep. Tetrahydrocannabivarin *(THCV)* is being studied for its potential role in appetite regulation and glycemic control.

These molecules often work better together, a concept known as the entourage effect. In many cases, whole-plant products provide broader benefit than isolated compounds alone.

Terpenes add another dimension: *linalool is linked to calm, beta-caryophyllene interacts with CB2 receptors to reduce inflammation, and pinene supports alertness and memory.* By adjusting cannabinoid ratios and terpene profiles, clinicians and patients can tailor Cannabis toward pain relief, sleep, focus, or mood support.

WHY THIS MATTERS

Cannabis in medicine is not a cultural experiment or a passing trend. It is an evidence-based therapy that deserves the same respect as any other treatment. For patients, it represents relief when pharmaceuticals fail or cause unbearable side effects. For doctors, it demands curiosity and ongoing education about the Endocannabinoid System, product selection, and dosing. For policymakers, it is a test of whether law will finally follow science and lived experience, rather than fear and stigma.

The cost of ignoring Cannabis in medicine has been high. Patients have suffered unnecessarily, research has been stalled, and lives have been shortened. Meanwhile, treatments with far greater risks such as opioids, benzodiazepines, and certain antidepressants became mainstream.

The lesson is clear: *prohibition did not protect health, it delayed progress.*

Cannabis is not simply another option. It is a reset button for how medicine views plants, patients, and science.

From here, we move through each condition. We will discuss pain, epilepsy, cancer, multiple sclerosis, mental health, and more. We will be guided by clarity, compassion, and a commitment to science.

Cannabis is not a cure, but for millions it is the difference between suffering and function, between endurance and dignity.

MEDICAL APPLICATIONS: CORE HEALTH CONDITIONS

"Cannabis earns its place in medicine through data, outcomes, and responsible application, not belief or trend."

05

ALZHEIMER'S DISEASE & DEMENTIA

A GLOBAL CHALLENGE

Alzheimer's disease is the most common cause of dementia, affecting tens of millions of families worldwide. It reshapes memory, identity, and daily life. For those living with the condition, ordinary moments such as sharing a meal, recognizing a face, or enjoying a quiet evening can become uncertain or disappear altogether. For caregivers, the demands are constant, often stretching emotional and physical endurance.

This is where Cannabis matters. Beyond politics and cultural debates, Cannabis has emerged as a tool for comfort, clarity, and connection. It does not promise a cure, but it can restore moments of peace, sleep, appetite, and calm.

These small victories add up: *a restful night after weeks of pacing, a full dinner shared without struggle, or a warm laugh at a familiar song.*

Around the world, from Israel to Canada, Europe to Australia, research and clinical programs are showing that Cannabis can transform the daily experience of Alzheimer's care.

THE ROLE OF THE ENDOCANNABINOID SYSTEM

The Endocannabinoid System is central to understanding why Cannabis has such profound effects on Alzheimer's. This network regulates memory, mood, inflammation, and cellular balance. CB1 receptors are abundant in the hippocampus and cortex, regions that form and retrieve memories. CB2 receptors are found throughout the immune system and in brain microglia, where they regulate inflammation and clean up cellular waste.

In Alzheimer's, the Endocannabinoid System takes on an even more important role. Neuroinflammation, oxidative stress, and toxic protein buildup place immense pressure on brain cells. Endocannabinoids act as modulators, calming excessive immune activity, supporting mitochondrial energy, and encouraging new connections between neurons. When cannabinoids from the plant interact with this system, they strengthen the body's natural balancing efforts. THC gently adjusts memory and mood signaling, while CBD reinforces calm, focus, and resilience against stress.

LABORATORY AND ANIMAL EVIDENCE

Decades of laboratory and animal studies provide a strong foundation for what families now witness in daily life. In cultured neurons, THC reduces the accumulation of amyloid beta, a hallmark of Alzheimer's pathology, while also improving synaptic signaling. CBD demonstrates powerful antioxidant activity, reducing oxidative stress and preserving mitochondrial energy.

In animal models, balanced cannabinoid formulations have improved performance on memory tasks, increased synaptic plasticity, and reduced neuroinflammation. In aging mice, low doses of THC restored learning ability and strengthened neural connections, suggesting that cannabinoids can support brain plasticity even later in life. CBD consistently reduces markers of inflammation and stabilizes mood and behavior in dementia models. These findings provide scientific confidence that what patients and caregivers describe has measurable biological roots.

HUMAN RESEARCH AND CLINICAL EXPERIENCE

Clinical programs around the world have extended these laboratory findings into patient care. Israel has been a leader, integrating Cannabis into geriatric and memory care. Studies document reduced agitation, better sleep, and improved appetite. Nurses report calmer evenings, smoother routines, and patients who are more engaged during the day.

In Canada, Cannabis is used in long-term care facilities with structured evening dosing to ease sundowning and nighttime restlessness.

Families often describe this as a return of peace to the household. In Europe, particularly in Germany, the Netherlands, and Spain, observational studies show that Cannabis oils and capsules improve caregiver burden and reduce behavioral disturbances. Australia has launched pilot programs focusing on CBD-rich formulations, finding improvements in agitation, mood stability, and quality of life.

One caregiver in Canada described how her husband, who had not slept through the night in years, finally rested peacefully after receiving evening Cannabis oil. *"It felt like I had my partner back, if only for a night,"* she said.

These experiences highlight what the data makes clear: *patients become more comfortable, caregivers feel supported, and daily life becomes more manageable and dignified.*

THERAPEUTIC TARGETS

Cannabis influences several processes in Alzheimer's disease at the same time. CBD and beta-caryophyllene calm overactive immune cells and reduce inflammatory cascades. Antioxidant activity from both CBD and THC helps preserve cellular energy and limit damage. Laboratory studies suggest cannabinoids may reduce the buildup of amyloid beta and tau proteins, easing stress on neurons.

By modulating neurotransmitters such as glutamate and GABA, cannabinoids encourage more balanced communication between brain cells. Through CB1 receptors in mood-regulating regions, cannabinoids reduce anxiety, agitation, and irritability, bringing comfort to patients and caregivers alike.

This broad activity explains why Cannabis feels so effective for multiple symptoms. It is not targeting a single receptor or pathway, but instead supporting balance across interconnected systems.

DAILY LIFE OUTCOMES

For families, science matters, but lived experience matters even more. Cannabis brings visible and meaningful changes. Meals become easier as appetite improves. Evenings calm as sundowning and pacing lessen. Nights grow more restful, reducing exhaustion for both patient and caregiver.

Caregivers describe subtle but powerful shifts: *a father humming to an old song, a grandmother enjoying dessert with a smile, or a spouse sleeping peacefully after months of restlessness.*

These moments restore dignity, strengthen bonds, and remind families of the person they love.

FORMULATIONS AND DELIVERY APPROACHES

Different formulations meet different needs in daily practice. Balanced oils with both THC and CBD are common in evening care, easing agitation and promoting sleep. CBD-forward oils or capsules are favored during the day to promote calm focus without intoxication. Tinctures allow flexible dosing and are often timed with meals or bedtime. Capsules provide consistency and predictability, helping caregivers follow a simple schedule. Topical products can ease stiffness that makes dressing or bathing more difficult.

Clinics and memory care programs often recommend establishing a daily rhythm of consistent meals, light activity, and scheduled Cannabis support, so the body and mind can settle into dependable patterns.

TERPENES AND MINOR CANNABINOIDS

The entourage of plant compounds enriches therapeutic effects. Linalool provides gentle calm and mood support.

Beta-caryophyllene interacts with CB2 receptors, reinforcing anti-inflammatory action. Pinene offers daytime alertness and memory support. CBG shows neuroprotective promise, while CBN contributes to nighttime relaxation. By selecting formulations that emphasize these molecules, patients and caregivers often find smoother and more comprehensive relief.

CAREGIVER PERSPECTIVES AND CARE MODELS

Across the world, caregivers and clinicians are developing care models that integrate Cannabis into daily routines. In Israel, evening

Cannabis oil is incorporated into nursing routines to ease evening agitation and promote calmer nights. In Canada, long-term care homes align Cannabis dosing with meals and music therapy to create calmer evenings. In Europe and Australia, families are given guidance on timing, ratios, and delivery methods, reducing stress and uncertainty.

Caregivers consistently report that their loved ones are more comfortable and engaged, households are calmer, and they themselves feel more rested and supported. In this way, Cannabis becomes more than a treatment, it becomes a partner in caregiving.

THE FUTURE OF RESEARCH

Research momentum continues to build. Scientists are mapping how cannabinoids influence synaptic plasticity, neurogenesis, and brain clearance systems. Clinical trials are testing morning and evening dosing protocols, balancing CBD during the day with gentle THC support at night. International collaborations are expanding, with Israel, Canada, the Netherlands, Spain, the United Kingdom, and Australia sharing data and harmonizing approaches.

Each study, each clinical program, and each family story contributes to a growing global understanding: *Cannabis has an essential role in the compassionate care of Alzheimer's and dementia.*

WHERE AMERICA HAS FALLEN BEHIND

While countries like Israel, Canada, and Germany have built structured programs around Cannabis and dementia care, the United States has struggled under outdated policies. For decades, Cannabis was locked in the most restrictive federal category, officially labeled as having no medical use. This designation blocked funding, slowed innovation, and prevented researchers from gathering the very evidence policymakers demanded.

Families in America were told there was not enough research, while at the same time policies made that research nearly impossible. Care homes and hospitals could not integrate Cannabis into care without risking federal penalties, even as colleagues overseas published studies and shared protocols.

The result is clear. Patients and families in the United States have waited longer for access, education, and guidance. Doctors and nurses have lacked training on the Endocannabinoid System, despite its relevance to memory, mood, and inflammation. The absence of funding and clinical trials slowed American medicine, while other countries raced ahead.

The opportunity now is to learn from this gap. By removing Cannabis from restrictive categories and investing in medical education, the United States can begin to close the distance. The science has never been in doubt, only the policies have. With barriers lifting, American patients and caregivers can finally benefit from the progress flourishing abroad. The cost of delay is measured not only in lost research years but in human suffering that could have been eased sooner.

WHY THIS MATTERS

Alzheimer's is one of the most difficult challenges a family can face. Cannabis offers a way to make days smoother, nights calmer, and connections stronger. It supports the body's balancing system, restores appetite, calms restlessness, and nurtures dignity.

For patients, this matters because moments of identity and connection can be preserved, whether that means sharing a meal, smiling at a cherished song, or sleeping peacefully through the night. For caregivers, this matters because Cannabis reduces agitation and strain, making the care journey less exhausting and more sustainable. Families often describe feeling like they can breathe again, knowing their loved one is calmer and more comfortable.

From a global perspective, this matters because research from Israel, Canada, Europe, and Australia consistently confirms the same truth: *Cannabis improves agitation, sleep, appetite, and mood.*

It has moved from anecdote to evidence, from taboo to trusted therapy. From a future perspective, this matters because Cannabis represents more than symptom management. It signals a shift toward therapies that honor the body's own systems and the whole person, rather than isolated symptoms.

This chapter is both a guide and a promise.

The guide is practical: *how Cannabis can be used, what outcomes to expect, and what families around the world are experiencing.*

The promise is hopeful: *with clear education and compassionate care, Cannabis will continue to transform Alzheimer's care, creating a legacy of brighter days and gentler nights for generations to come.*

06

EPILEPSY & SEIZURES

A GLOBAL BURDEN

Epilepsy is one of the most common neurological conditions in the world, affecting nearly fifty-million people across every continent. For one-third of these patients, standard medications do not provide seizure control. The impact extends far beyond the seizures themselves. Families live with constant fear of the next episode, children miss school and important developmental milestones, and adults struggle with independence and employment. The weight of epilepsy is carried not only by the individual with the condition but also by everyone who loves and supports them.

Cannabis has emerged as a powerful ally in this space. While it is not a cure, it has proven to be a tool that brings relief, restores quality of life, and offers families hope. The story of Cannabis and epilepsy is one of science, compassion, and global cooperation.

HOW CANNABIS INTERACTS WITH THE BRAIN

The discovery of the Endocannabinoid System helped explain why Cannabis plays such an important role in seizure control. CB1 receptors are abundant in brain regions involved in memory, movement, and electrical signaling, including the hippocampus and cortex. When brain networks become overexcited, seizures occur. The Endocannabinoid System acts like a stabilizer, calming overactivity and restoring balance.

CBD does not cause intoxication and has become the focus of epilepsy research worldwide. It works across multiple pathways at once. CBD indirectly modulates CB1 receptors, calms excitatory signals through TRPV1 channels, interacts with GPR55 to reduce overactivity, and supports adenosine signaling, helping restore calm to the brain's circuits. This multilayered approach is why CBD is often described as a circuit breaker, preventing runaway electrical storms that produce seizures.

BREAKTHROUGH CASES AND AWARENESS

The modern movement began with a young girl named Charlotte Figi, who lived with Dravet syndrome, a rare and severe form of epilepsy. Traditional medicines had failed, and her family turned to a CBD-rich extract. Her seizures, which had numbered in the hundreds each week, dropped dramatically. For the first time in years, Charlotte smiled, played, and connected with her family.

Her story captured worldwide attention and inspired the Realm of Caring Foundation, which now supports thousands of families exploring Cannabis therapies for epilepsy. Charlotte's journey showed the world that Cannabis was not simply an alternative idea but a life-changing medicine. Similar stories soon emerged in Israel, Canada, and Europe, where families reported children returning to school, regaining milestones, and enjoying childhood again.

CLINICAL TRIALS AND STRONGEST EVIDENCE

The individual stories were powerful, but they were soon supported by rigorous science. Randomized controlled trials published in journals such as *The New England Journal of Medicine* and *The Lancet Neurology* confirmed what families had been reporting. In children with Dravet syndrome, Lennox-Gastaut syndrome, and tuberous sclerosis complex, CBD oils reduced seizure frequency by 40-50 percent compared with placebo. In some children, seizures were reduced by 70 percent or more.

These trials measured not only seizure counts but also quality of life. Parents reported better sleep, improved mood, and enhanced overall functioning. In medical language, the results were significant. In family language, the results were transformative.

FDA-APPROVED CBD AND PRACTICAL USE

In 2018, the United States Food and Drug Administration approved Epidiolex, a purified CBD oil, for severe childhood epilepsies. This was the first Cannabis-derived medicine to achieve federal approval in the United States. It validated decades of patient advocacy and international research.

Families describe beginning with low daily doses, gradually building to the ranges studied in clinical trials. Results are often seen within weeks, with reductions in seizures, improved alertness, and renewed engagement in school and play. The approval encouraged more physicians to learn about Cannabis therapies and to guide families with confidence.

GLOBAL PROGRAMS BEYOND THE FDA

Other countries moved even more quickly. Israel created structured pediatric programs where Cannabis oils are monitored and adjusted under medical supervision. Canadian families accessed Cannabis therapies nationally with physician oversight and pharmacy support. In Europe, particularly in Germany and Spain, observational studies showed reductions in seizures and improvements in family well-being. Australia established pediatric neurology programs that integrate Cannabis into clinical care, with government-backed registries tracking outcomes.

The consistency of findings across continents is striking. No matter the country or the program, Cannabis oils brought seizure relief, calmer routines, and renewed hope.

REAL-WORLD DATA AND PATIENT EXPERIENCES

Numbers and trials are important, but lived experience is what families remember most. Parents describe fewer emergency visits, children sleeping through the night for the first time in years, and siblings finally able to play without constant fear.

Registries in Israel and Canada confirm these impressions. Thousands of families report not only seizure reduction but also improvements in behavior, communication, and daily function.

Caregivers often say the most powerful change is simple: *they feel they have their child back.*

One mother described how her son, who had been unable to attend school because of constant seizures, returned to the classroom after beginning CBD oil. She said the joy of packing his backpack in the morning felt like a miracle.

WHOLE PLANT VS. PURIFIED CBD

While purified CBD oils such as Epidiolex have proven effective, many families prefer whole-plant extracts. These contain CBD along with small amounts of THC, other cannabinoids, and terpenes. The synergy among these compounds is often called the entourage effect.

Terpenes add additional benefits. Linalool contributes calming qualities. Myrcene supports rest and relaxation. Beta-caryophyllene interacts with CB2 receptors to reduce inflammation. For some families, these broader formulations provide smoother results with fewer breakthrough seizures. The variety of approaches allows medicine to be personalized to each child's needs.

OTHER CANNABINOIDS AND FUTURE DIRECTIONS

The research horizon continues to expand. Cannabidiolic acid *(CBDA)* has shown strong anti-seizure potential in preclinical models. Tetrahydrocannabinolic acid *(THCA)* is being studied for neuroprotective qualities. Minor cannabinoids such as CBG and CBN are also being explored as supportive options.

The future of Cannabis in epilepsy care will likely involve tailored blends of cannabinoids and terpenes designed for specific seizure types. Research is accelerating, and international cooperation is helping unlock the full potential of the plant.

CAREGIVER PERSPECTIVES AND PRACTICAL GUIDANCE

For caregivers, Cannabis brings relief in more ways than one. Fewer seizures mean more school days attended, more play dates kept, and more time for siblings to simply be children. Families describe new routines with CBD or balanced oils that are simple, repeatable, and effective.

Tinctures provide flexible dosing, capsules bring consistency, and sprays can be used for urgent relief.

Caregivers often emphasize not just the medical outcomes but the emotional transformation: *a calmer household, restored confidence, and renewed energy for parents who no longer live in constant fear.*

For many, Cannabis means hope restored.

POLICY AND RESEARCH NEEDS

The momentum is unstoppable. As more countries see the benefits, barriers are falling. Laws are changing, funding is opening, and researchers are collaborating across borders. The next steps are broader trials, long-term studies, and insurance coverage to make Cannabis therapies accessible to every family in need. This is not a question of *if*, but *when*. The evidence has already shown that Cannabis helps epilepsy.

In the United States, however, families were often forced to uproot and move to states with legal programs, or risk breaking federal law, to access life-changing therapies. This injustice slowed adoption and left countless children without relief while other countries advanced. The cost was measured in missed milestones and preventable suffering.

WHY THIS MATTERS

Epilepsy is not just seizures. It is lost moments, interrupted childhoods, exhausted parents, and families stretched to the limit.

Cannabis changes this story. It brings peace where there was chaos, sleep where there was fear, and hope where there was despair.

But this is not only about families in one city or one country. Around the world, access to Cannabis can mean the difference between children who learn, laugh, and grow, and children who remain trapped in cycles of suffering. In Israel, Canada, and parts of Europe, families find relief with structured medical programs. In other places, the same families risk prison, financial ruin, or hopelessness for trying to save their children.

This global imbalance is not science; it is policy.

It reveals a hard truth: *justice in health care is not evenly distributed.*

That is why this story must become a call to action. Doctors must be willing to learn, lawmakers must be willing to listen, and communities must be willing to stand with families who are fighting for care. Every seizure prevented is not only a medical achievement, it is a restored childhood, a renewed marriage, a parent who can finally exhale.

These victories should not depend on ZIP codes, wealth, or political winds.

This chapter is also part of a larger truth. For decades, prohibition clouded judgment and delayed science, while patients and caregivers proved the truth in real time. Epilepsy has shown the world what is possible when fear gives way to compassion and evidence. To clear the smoke is to do more than correct mistakes of the past; it is to promise a future where no family is left behind in the dark.

The evidence has already shown that Cannabis helps epilepsy.

07

CHRONIC PAIN

A GLOBAL BURDEN

Chronic pain is one of the most widespread health problems in the world. It affects daily function, mental health, and quality of life for millions. For decades, treatment has centered on opioids and other drugs that carry significant risks. Cannabis has emerged as a promising alternative, attracting interest from researchers and patients alike. Unlike therapies that only mask symptoms temporarily, Cannabis interacts with the body's own balancing system, offering both relief and restoration.

HOW THE ENDOCANNABINOID SYSTEM CONNECTS TO PAIN

The Endocannabinoid System is deeply involved in regulating pain. CB1 receptors in the brain and spinal cord limit the intensity of pain signals, while CB2 receptors in the immune system help reduce inflammation that fuels chronic pain. Endocannabinoids also influence serotonin and dopamine, supporting mood and resilience in patients who struggle with the emotional burden of pain. TRPV1 channels, another target of cannabinoids, play a direct role in neuropathic pain and are calmed when Cannabis compounds interact with them.

This broad interaction explains why cannabinoids may benefit such a wide range of conditions, from nerve damage to arthritis. For some patients, Cannabis does more than quiet the signal of pain. It alters how the body responds, calming overactive pathways and reducing the inflammation that drives them.

WHAT THE RESEARCH SHOWS

Evidence has steadily grown over the past two decades. In 2007, a United States study published in *Neurology* found that smoked Cannabis reduced neuropathic pain in patients with HIV by about one-third, with no serious adverse effects. A follow-up trial in 2009 confirmed these results, and by 2013 a California study showed that vaporized Cannabis provided meaningful relief with minimal cognitive side effects.

Beyond neuropathy, musculoskeletal and inflammatory pain have also been studied. In 2006, a United Kingdom trial of an oromucosal THC and CBD spray in rheumatoid arthritis patients showed reduced pain during movement and improved sleep. Canadian researchers later investigated fibromyalgia, reporting that synthetic cannabinoids improved pain, sleep quality, and overall quality of life compared with placebo.

Headaches and migraines are another area of growing research. In 2024, a United States crossover trial tested vaporized Cannabis with balanced THC and CBD. Patients experienced significant improvements in migraine relief compared with placebo, reinforcing decades of patient testimony that Cannabis can stop or soften attacks where conventional medicines fail.

CONDITION SPECIFIC EXAMPLES

Diabetic neuropathy: *Patients often report reduced burning pain and better sleep with balanced Cannabis oils.*

Arthritis: *THC and CBD sprays have improved mobility and reduced morning stiffness in trials, offering an option where standard anti-inflammatory drugs fail.*

Fibromyalgia: *Many patients describe Cannabis as the first therapy that touches both pain and sleep, consistent with the theory of clinical endocannabinoid deficiency.*

Migraines: *Patients often note faster relief from inhaled Cannabis compared with oral painkillers, reducing both intensity and duration of attacks.*

GENERALIZED CHRONIC PAIN

Not all patients can point to a single diagnosis. Many live with persistent, nonspecific pain that resists traditional explanations and treatments. For these individuals, Cannabis can still provide relief. By calming overactive pain pathways and improving sleep, it reduces the daily burden of discomfort even when no clear medical label exists. Patients often describe feeling more functional and more engaged in daily life, even if the source of their pain remains uncertain.

PATIENT OUTCOMES

Real world data confirms the clinical findings. Observational studies in Israel, Canada, and the United States show that many chronic pain patients report meaningful relief, better sleep, and reduced reliance on prescription drugs once Cannabis is introduced. Israeli registries covering thousands of patients reveal consistent reductions in pain scores and improvements in quality of life.

One patient in Toronto, who had lived with disabling back pain for years, described the change this way: *"For the first time in a decade, I was able to walk my dog without stopping every block to rest. It did not erase my pain completely, but it gave me my life back in a way no pill ever did."*

Stories like this echo across clinics worldwide, bringing human meaning to the statistics.

VETERANS AND PAIN RELIEF

Among veterans, chronic pain is one of the most common service-related conditions. Studies from the United States Department of Veterans Affairs estimate that nearly 60 percent of veterans returning from combat report persistent pain. Many are prescribed opioids, which often create dependency without lasting relief.

Cannabis offers another path. Surveys of veterans enrolled in state medical Cannabis programs show reductions in both pain intensity and opioid use. In one large survey, more than half of veteran participants reported that Cannabis allowed them to cut their opioid dose or stop it entirely. Beyond numbers, veterans describe being able to sleep through the night without heavy sedatives, to participate in family life without constant fog, and to feel more in control of their recovery.

ROUTES OF ADMINISTRATION AND PRACTICAL USE

Different formulations meet different needs. Inhaled Cannabis provides rapid relief for breakthrough pain or migraines. Oils and tinctures offer steady control for neuropathy and arthritis. Capsules bring consistency and are often used for long-term management. Topicals can ease localized pain such as arthritic joints or muscle injuries.

Terpenes add another dimension. Linalool supports calm and relaxation. Myrcene promotes rest. Beta-caryophyllene interacts with CB2 receptors to reinforce anti-inflammatory action. Pinene supports focus and clarity. By adjusting these profiles, Cannabis can be tailored to individual needs.

OPIOID REDUCTION AND PUBLIC HEALTH

Perhaps the most compelling reason to study Cannabis for chronic pain is its potential to reduce reliance on opioids. Opioids kill tens of thousands every year through overdose, while Cannabis has never caused a fatal overdose in recorded history. Multiple studies in the United States show that in states with medical Cannabis programs, opioid prescribing rates have declined. Some analyses also suggest lower overdose deaths in those states, though results vary by study design.

The consistent signal is clear: *Cannabis offers a safer option for many patients, one that may reduce exposure to the risks of long term opioid therapy.*

Chronic pain is not only a medical problem but also an economic and social one. It remains one of the leading causes of lost workdays, disability claims, and healthcare costs. By offering an alternative path to relief, Cannabis has the potential to ease the suffering of individuals while also reducing broader burdens on society.

WHY THIS MATTERS

Chronic pain affects millions and places a heavy burden on individuals, families, and healthcare systems. Current treatments are often inadequate, addictive, or unsafe over the long term. Cannabis is not a miracle cure, but it is supported by biology, clinical trials, and real world evidence. For patients who have exhausted conventional therapies, it may offer a pathway toward relief, function, and dignity.

This matters because every day lost to pain is a day taken from life itself. By restoring mobility, supporting sleep, and reducing dependence on dangerous opioids, Cannabis gives people back their routines, their relationships, and their hope. From a public health perspective, it could reduce overdose deaths, lower healthcare costs, and strengthen communities. From a human perspective, it turns survival into living again.

The future of pain management will not be written by opioids alone. It will be shaped by safer, smarter, and more compassionate therapies. Cannabis is at the center of that change.

08

CANCER (SYMPTOMS & SUPPORT)

CANCER AND THE BIRTH OF MEDICAL CANNABIS

Cancer is one of the most feared diagnoses in the world. In the United States it is the second leading cause of death, responsible for more than six hundred thousand deaths each year. Globally, more than ten million people die from cancer annually. Behind these numbers are families facing fear, uncertainty, and the heavy weight of treatment.

Cannabis became part of the cancer story long before legalization spread across the United States. In 1996 California passed Proposition 215, the first modern medical Cannabis law in the country. It was cancer patients who led that movement. They were not motivated by politics but by the need for relief. They sought dignity in the face of chemotherapy, appetite in the face of wasting, and rest in the face of sleepless nights. Their voices reshaped American medicine and began a global wave of change.

THE ENDOCANNABINOID SYSTEM AND CANCER SYMPTOMS

The Endocannabinoid System is central to how Cannabis helps people with cancer. CB1 receptors in the brain regulate nausea, appetite, and pain perception. CB2 receptors are found in the immune system and peripheral tissues, where they calm inflammation and support balance.

Cannabinoids from the plant interact with both sets of receptors, giving them a unique role in supportive oncology care. THC stimulates appetite, reduces nausea, and eases pain. CBD calms anxiety, supports sleep, and provides anti-inflammatory balance. Together, supported by terpenes and minor cannabinoids, Cannabis engages the body's own healing systems to bring relief across multiple symptoms.

NAUSEA AND VOMITING

Chemotherapy induced nausea and vomiting, often called *CINV*, is one of the most difficult parts of cancer treatment. For decades, patients turned to Cannabis when standard anti-nausea medications were not enough. In the 1980s the United States Food and Drug Administration approved synthetic THC medications such as dronabinol and nabilone for chemotherapy nausea. Yet patients often found that whole plant Cannabis worked better.

Patients describe being able to finish meals, tolerate chemotherapy, and even share laughter at the dinner table because Cannabis reduced their nausea. For many, this difference meant the ability to complete treatment without interruption. One woman in California described her experience this way: *"Cannabis was the only thing that let me eat with my grandchildren again."* For her, it was not simply relief from nausea but the return of family connection in the middle of treatment.

APPETITE AND CACHEXIA

Loss of appetite and weight loss, often called cachexia, are among the most devastating effects of cancer. Malnutrition weakens the body, reduces tolerance to treatment, and lowers quality of life. Cannabis restores appetite in a way that is both effective and enjoyable. Patients often describe food tasting better and meals becoming social again.

Registry data from Israel and surveys from Canada show consistent improvement in appetite and weight stabilization among cancer patients using Cannabis. Families tell stories of loved ones who return to the table, eat with enthusiasm, and regain strength. Something as simple as finishing dinner becomes a symbol of victory.

PAIN MANAGEMENT

Pain is one of the most common and distressing symptoms of cancer. It can arise from tumors pressing on nerves, bone metastases, surgery, or chemotherapy induced neuropathy. Traditional pain management often relies on opioids, which bring sedation and dependence.

Cannabis offers a different path. Clinical trials in the United Kingdom, Canada, and Israel have shown that Cannabis extracts reduce cancer related pain even in patients already using opioids. Balanced THC and CBD formulations help manage nerve pain, bone pain, and treatment related discomfort. Patients often report needing fewer opioids and experiencing clearer minds and better function.

For families, this means a parent or spouse who is awake, alert, and able to share conversation and connection without being dulled by heavy medication.

SLEEP, ANXIETY, AND EMOTIONAL BURDEN

Cancer is not only a physical disease but also an emotional journey. Anxiety, fear, and sleeplessness weigh heavily on patients and families. Cannabis provides relief across these domains. CBD calms anxiety and quiets racing thoughts. THC encourages deeper, more restorative sleep. Terpenes such as linalool and myrcene enhance relaxation and comfort.

Patients describe falling asleep more easily, staying asleep longer, and waking with less dread. Families often note that Cannabis brings back moments of laughter, calm evenings, and emotional resilience.

PALLIATIVE AND HOSPICE CARE

In the final stages of cancer, the goals of care shift from cure to comfort. Cannabis plays a profound role here. It eases pain, restores appetite, and brings rest. For many patients it allows time with family to be marked not by struggle but by peace.

In Israel, Cannabis is integrated into hospice protocols, where patients and families consistently report greater comfort and dignity. In the United States, hospices in states with medical Cannabis programs describe patients resting more peacefully and caregivers feeling more supported. Cannabis, at life's end, becomes not just a medicine but a companion for dignity.

REAL WORLD DATA AND GLOBAL PROGRAMS

The global evidence is remarkably consistent. In Israel, national registries track thousands of cancer patients using Cannabis, with improvements in pain, appetite, and quality of life. In Canada, palliative care centers integrate Cannabis into treatment plans, reducing reliance on opioids and improving family satisfaction. In Europe, countries such as Germany, Spain, and the Netherlands have expanded access for oncology patients with strong outcomes.

In the United States progress has been uneven due to federal restrictions, but patient voices remain strong. Across dozens of states, cancer patients report that Cannabis makes the difference between enduring treatment and living through it with dignity.

FORMULATIONS AND DELIVERY

Different symptoms call for different approaches. Oils and tinctures provide steady support for pain and appetite. Vaporization offers rapid relief for sudden nausea. Capsules deliver consistent dosing for daily management. Topicals soothe localized pain from tumors or surgical scars. Balanced THC and CBD formulations help with both physical and emotional symptoms.

Terpenes provide additional nuance. Linalool supports calm, myrcene promotes rest, and beta-caryophyllene reduces inflammation. Patients and caregivers often develop daily routines timed with meals and rest, bringing predictability and comfort.

CAREGIVER AND FAMILY PERSPECTIVES

Cancer affects the entire household. Caregivers carry the emotional weight of watching loved ones struggle. When Cannabis brings appetite, sleep, or laughter back into the home, the relief spreads to the whole family.

Parents describe the joy of seeing a child with cancer eat ice cream again. Spouses share the comfort of sleeping side by side through the night. Children of older adults speak of treasured conversations in peaceful moments. Cannabis helps restore connection, which is often the most important medicine of all.

POLICY AND RESEARCH NEEDS

Cancer patients were pioneers of the modern medical Cannabis movement. Their voices and advocacy brought legalization to the United States and inspired the world. The need for expanded research is clear. While Israel, Canada, and Europe lead with national programs and clinical trials, the United States still faces barriers that limit progress.

Federal scheduling labeled Cannabis as a substance with no medical use for decades, even as patients demonstrated the opposite. This mismatch delayed innovation, left doctors without education, and forced patients to navigate inconsistent laws. It was not science that held Cannabis back in oncology care, it was stigma and policy.

The opportunity now is to honor the legacy of cancer patients by advancing research, education, and access. With every new study and every new patient story, the case becomes stronger. Cannabis must be part of standard oncology care.

WHY THIS MATTERS

Cancer is one of humanity's greatest challenges. It disrupts bodies, families, and communities. The symptoms it brings, pain, nausea, loss of appetite, exhaustion, and fear, are overwhelming. Cannabis addresses these burdens with compassion and effectiveness.

This matters because cancer patients built the foundation of the medical Cannabis movement. Their demand for dignity created the first laws in California and sparked a global wave of acceptance. It matters because every meal finished, every night of sleep restored, and every laugh shared is a victory. Each small win lightens the weight of disease.

Cannabis does more than ease symptoms. It restores humanity in the face of one of life's hardest battles. It brings peace to patients, strength to caregivers, and hope to families. For the United States and the world, Cannabis in cancer care is not just an option, it is an essential act of compassion born from the voices of those who needed it most.

This chapter is a reminder that policy debates and scientific details are not abstractions, they are about real people. When a mother can hold down food again, when a father can sleep through the night, when a child can share one more laugh with a parent, those are victories that matter more than statistics. Cannabis makes those victories possible, and that is why it must remain at the heart of compassionate care.

Cannabis does more than ease symptoms; it restores humanity in the face of one of life's hardest battles.

09

FIBROMYALGIA

UNDERSTANDING FIBROMYALGIA

Fibromyalgia is a chronic condition that affects an estimated four million adults in the United States and millions more worldwide. It is marked by widespread pain, profound fatigue, sleep disruption, and cognitive issues often called fibro fog. For those who live with it, daily life can feel unpredictable and overwhelming. Some mornings begin with stiffness that makes it hard to get out of bed. Others are clouded by fatigue so heavy that even routine tasks feel impossible.

What makes fibromyalgia especially difficult is that it is an invisible illness. There are no outward signs, no blood tests, and no scans that confirm its presence. Patients often spend years seeking answers, moving from doctor to doctor, sometimes doubted or dismissed. Families, workplaces, and communities struggle to understand what they cannot see. The emotional toll is heavy, and many feel isolated in their suffering.

THE ENDOCANNABINOID SYSTEM AND FIBROMYALGIA

The Endocannabinoid System is the body's own balancing network, regulating pain, mood, sleep, and immune activity. For fibromyalgia patients, this system seems to be out of alignment. One leading theory is called clinical endocannabinoid deficiency.

It proposes that conditions like fibromyalgia, migraines, and irritable bowel syndrome share a common thread: *not enough endocannabinoid activity to maintain normal balance.*

Cannabinoids from the plant appear to fill this gap. THC interacts with CB1 receptors in the nervous system, calming the overactive pain signals that make fibromyalgia so debilitating. CBD interacts with multiple pathways, easing anxiety, lifting mood, and supporting restorative sleep. Together, they help restore the volume control of the nervous system, quieting its constant and excessive alarms.

RESEARCH EVIDENCE AROUND THE WORLD

Scientific evidence for Cannabis and fibromyalgia is steadily growing, with promising results from many countries.

In Canada, small clinical trials with nabilone, a synthetic cannabinoid, showed improvements in pain, sleep quality, and overall patient well being.

In Spain, an observational study of fibromyalgia patients found that Cannabis use led to reductions in pain and stiffness, along with improved relaxation, mood, and perception of well being. Patients reported that their quality of life improved dramatically.

Israel, a global leader in medical Cannabis, has included fibromyalgia in its national program for years. Registry data covering hundreds of patients shows meaningful reductions in pain, better sleep, and reductions in the use of opioids and other prescription drugs.

In the United States, patient surveys reveal similar patterns. Many report reducing or eliminating prescription pain medications, antidepressants, and sleep aids. Advocacy groups have been critical in pushing for recognition of fibromyalgia as a qualifying condition in state medical Cannabis programs.

Across Europe, Germany and the Netherlands have integrated Cannabis into pain clinics, with fibromyalgia patients among the most common recipients.

In Australia, prescription data shows fibromyalgia as one of the top conditions for which medical Cannabis is prescribed, reflecting both need and success.

The message from every region is consistent: *Cannabis works where other treatments have failed.*

HOW CANNABIS HELPS WITH CORE SYMPTOMS

Pain: *By modulating CB1 and CB2 receptors, Cannabis reduces the intensity of widespread musculoskeletal pain. Patients describe the constant ache softening and becoming more manageable.*

Sleep: *THC supports sleep onset, while CBD calms anxiety that often disrupts the night. Patients often report sleeping more deeply and waking more refreshed.*

Fatigue: *While Cannabis does not directly treat fatigue, the improvements in sleep and pain reduce exhaustion, allowing patients to regain energy.*

Mood and Anxiety: *CBD-rich formulations bring calm and stability. THC in low doses can lift mood and reduce tension. Together they help soften the emotional weight of fibromyalgia.*

Cognitive Function: *With pain and anxiety reduced, many patients report clearer thinking and less fibro fog.*

This multi-symptom approach is what makes Cannabis unique. It does not target just one aspect of fibromyalgia but brings relief across the whole spectrum of suffering.

REAL WORLD DATA AND PATIENT VOICES

Clinical studies provide data, but patient voices bring the story to life. Many describe Cannabis as the first treatment that gave them back a sense of normalcy. Some say it is the first time in years they have slept through the night. Others tell of finally being able to cook, clean, or walk without overwhelming pain.

One patient described Cannabis as the first thing that allowed her to cook dinner and eat with her family again without collapsing from pain. For her, Cannabis was not simply relief, it was restoration of daily life.

Families notice the difference too. A parent can once again play with their child. A partner can once again share a walk or a meal without being cut short by exhaustion. Caregivers feel relief as the household regains rhythm and joy.

Registry data from Israel, Canada, and the United States confirms these experiences. Patients consistently report lower pain scores, better mood, and fewer medications. For many, Cannabis is not simply an option. It is the first therapy that made them feel human again.

FORMULATIONS AND APPROACHES

Fibromyalgia patients often experiment with different Cannabis formulations until they find what works best. Oils and tinctures are commonly used for steady relief throughout the day. Vaporization offers rapid control of flare ups when pain becomes severe. Topical creams and balms provide localized relief for tender points and sore muscles. Capsules allow consistent dosing and make daily routines easier.

Balanced THC and CBD ratios are often preferred, though some rely more on CBD during the day for clarity and THC at night for rest. Terpenes define the character and direction of each approach. Linalool enhances calm and relaxation. Myrcene supports restful sleep. Beta-caryophyllene interacts with CB2 receptors to reduce inflammation. Patients describe these combinations as smoothing out the effects, making relief more complete and predictable.

GLOBAL AND UNITED STATES PERSPECTIVES

Globally, countries like Israel and Canada are far ahead in structured fibromyalgia research and care. Their national programs collect data, guide dosing, and refine best practices. In Europe, fibromyalgia patients are included in pain management registries, and access is expanding as more evidence emerges. Australia continues to grow its national prescribing system, with fibromyalgia consistently listed among top conditions.

In the United States, progress has been uneven. Federal restrictions limit large clinical trials, but state programs have opened the door. Patients across many states now have access to Cannabis for fibromyalgia, though coverage and access remain inconsistent.

This mismatch is not scientific, it is political. Fibromyalgia patients have long been told their suffering was not real. Federal barriers repeated that same dismissal by slowing research and denying access. It was stigma and policy, not science, that held progress back.

Fibromyalgia patients have become some of the strongest voices in the medical Cannabis movement. Their persistence has helped reshape laws, destigmatize treatment, and expand access for millions of others.

WHY THIS MATTERS

Fibromyalgia is an illness that too often leaves people feeling invisible, doubted, and dismissed. For decades, patients were told that little could be done, or that the problem was in their heads. Meanwhile, they endured relentless pain, fatigue, and loss of quality of life.

Cannabis changes that story. It validates their experience and provides real relief. It allows patients to sleep, to think clearly, and to move with less pain. It restores dignity and makes everyday life possible again.

This matters because fibromyalgia is more than an individual struggle. It is a family struggle, a workplace struggle, and a societal struggle. When patients are restored, households heal, workplaces gain back productivity, and communities gain back members who can contribute fully.

For the United States and the world, embracing Cannabis for fibromyalgia is an act of compassion and progress. It acknowledges suffering that has been ignored and offers a solution that restores lives.

It also honors the voices of fibromyalgia patients themselves, who became advocates not just for their own relief but for broader recognition of Cannabis in medicine. Their persistence has shaped laws, guided research priorities, and given voice to invisible illnesses everywhere.

Cannabis is not just a treatment for fibromyalgia. It is a turning point for how we care for invisible illnesses, reminding the world that dignity and compassion are essential in every corner of medicine.

10

MULTIPLE SCLEROSIS

UNDERSTANDING MULTIPLE SCLEROSIS

Multiple sclerosis, often called MS, is a chronic autoimmune disease that attacks the protective covering of nerves known as myelin. When the immune system mistakenly targets these tissues, the nervous system is disrupted, leading to a wide range of symptoms. For some, the disease progresses slowly with long periods of stability. For others, symptoms arrive in sharp relapses and worsen quickly.

In the United States, nearly one million people live with MS. Symptoms include spasticity, muscle stiffness, neuropathic pain, fatigue, tremors, bladder and bowel dysfunction, mobility challenges, and cognitive decline.

The condition affects not only the patient but also their family and caregivers. It can reshape daily life, transforming simple tasks such as dressing, walking, or preparing meals into exhausting challenges. Emotional stress, loss of independence, and financial burdens weigh heavily on households.

THE ENDOCANNABINOID SYSTEM AND MS

The Endocannabinoid System is deeply connected to the biology of MS. CB1 receptors, found in the brain and spinal cord, regulate motor control, spasticity, and coordination. CB2 receptors, present in immune cells, help regulate inflammation. Because MS involves both nervous system disruption and immune system overreaction, Cannabis is uniquely suited to address it.

THC interacts with CB1 receptors, calming overactive motor circuits, reducing spasms, and easing neuropathic pain. CBD modulates inflammation through CB2 pathways, reduces anxiety, and supports cognition. Together, cannabinoids balance nervous system signaling and immune system activity, addressing the dual nature of MS in a way few other medicines can.

THE UNITED STATES PERSPECTIVE

MS is recognized as a qualifying condition in most state medical Cannabis programs. Patients with MS were among the earliest advocates for legalization, and their stories helped shift public opinion. Surveys by the National Multiple Sclerosis Society show that thousands of patients already use Cannabis, with the majority reporting improvements in pain, sleep, and spasticity.

While federal law still restricts large clinical trials, smaller US studies have confirmed benefits for muscle stiffness, spasms, and pain. Patients in states with access describe improvements in mobility, independence, and emotional well-being. Veterans with MS often note that Cannabis eases not only their neurological symptoms but also the anxiety and insomnia that come with chronic illness.

Yet the United States continues to lag behind global leaders in research. This is not because of lack of science but because of policy and stigma. Federal scheduling blocks progress, even as patients demonstrate benefits every day. MS patients remain advocates at the front lines, pushing lawmakers to catch up with both evidence and human need.

RESEARCH EVIDENCE AROUND THE WORLD

Globally, research on Cannabis for MS is among the most advanced of any medical condition. In the United Kingdom, nabiximols, an oromucosal spray containing THC and CBD, has been approved for MS spasticity since 2010. Clinical trials demonstrated meaningful improvements in muscle stiffness, mobility, and quality of sleep. Canada, Spain, and Germany followed with approvals, supported by observational data that confirmed sustained benefits.

Israel has conducted extensive research showing that Cannabis improves neuropathic pain, spasticity, bladder function, and sleep in MS patients. Italian studies found similar results, particularly in reducing neuropathic pain that resists traditional medication. In Australia, prescribing data shows MS as one of the most common neurological conditions treated with Cannabis.

The consistency across countries is striking. No matter the region, Cannabis improves quality of life for MS patients, often in ways that standard treatments cannot.

SYMPTOM RELIEF IN DAILY LIFE

One of the most widely reported benefits of Cannabis in MS is relief from spasticity. THC reduces stiffness and painful muscle spasms, allowing patients to move more freely and with less fear of sudden immobilization.

Neuropathic pain, which is often resistant to conventional medications, also responds to Cannabis. Both THC and CBD have shown effectiveness in easing this type of pain, giving patients an option when standard treatments fail.

Sleep disturbances, which plague many people with MS, often improve with balanced Cannabis formulations. Patients report deeper, more restorative rest that supports energy and function during the day.

Bladder dysfunction is another symptom where patients describe improvements. Nighttime interruptions decrease, and daytime control improves, which restores confidence and makes public life easier.

Cannabis also touches mood and cognition. CBD-rich formulations reduce anxiety and stabilize mood, while balanced cannabinoid ratios support clearer thinking. The result is not only physical relief but also improved emotional stability and cognitive function.

These improvements are not just clinical markers. They are life changing experiences. Being able to walk across a room without collapsing, sleeping through the night without interruption, or enjoying a conversation without constant distraction can transform a patient's daily life.

PATIENT OUTCOMES AND QUALITY OF LIFE

The most important outcome of Cannabis use in MS is independence. Patients describe regaining the ability to dress without exhaustion, rest without constant pain, and walk without unrelenting spasticity. For many, Cannabis makes the difference between living in isolation and actively participating in family life, contributing at work, or returning to hobbies once thought impossible.

One patient described Cannabis as the difference between needing a wheelchair full-time and being able to walk short distances with support. For that patient, Cannabis represented freedom and dignity, not simply symptom relief.

Families notice the ripple effect. When MS symptoms are controlled, caregivers sleep better, households function more smoothly, and emotional tension eases. Cannabis restores not just physical ability but also dignity, relationships, and joy.

FORMULATIONS AND APPROACHES

Different Cannabis formulations offer flexibility for managing MS. Oromucosal sprays such as nabiximols are widely used in Europe and Canada for spasticity. Oils and tinctures provide steady relief across the day, while vaporization offers rapid relief during sudden spasms or flare-ups. Capsules ensure consistent daily dosing, while topicals are used to soothe localized muscle and joint pain.

Terpenes refine these formulations, shaping their tone and effect. Linalool supports calm, myrcene promotes restful sleep, and beta-caryophyllene reduces inflammation. By tailoring ratios of cannabinoids and terpenes, patients can find formulations that match their individual needs.

GLOBAL COMPARISONS

MS patients worldwide have benefited from structured Cannabis programs for more than a decade. The United Kingdom, Germany, Spain, and Canada have approved Cannabis sprays as standard therapies. Israel continues to lead in research and patient registries, producing some of the most detailed long-term data available.

Australia's national system is expanding quickly, with MS consistently among the top conditions treated.

The United States has been slower, limited by federal restrictions, but patient demand has made MS a recognized condition in most state programs. The future lies in harmonizing United States policy with global progress so that American patients can benefit from the same structured care as those abroad.

WHY THIS MATTERS

MS is a disease that robs people of independence, mobility, and daily joy. It disrupts families, careers, and identities. Cannabis does more than reduce symptoms. It restores the ability to walk, to sleep, to laugh, and to connect. It gives families back their rhythm and patients back their dignity.

This matters because MS patients were among the pioneers of the medical Cannabis movement. Their advocacy helped legalize programs across the United States and beyond. It matters because Cannabis addresses multiple disabling symptoms at once, something few other treatments can achieve.

For the United States, expanding research and access means more than aligning with global progress. It means honoring the voices of patients who demanded relief and built the foundation of modern medical Cannabis. Their courage gave legitimacy to the movement worldwide. For families living with MS, Cannabis is not just medicine. It is a lifeline to independence, dignity, and hope.

11

PARKINSON'S DISEASE

UNDERSTANDING PARKINSON'S DISEASE

Parkinson's disease is a progressive neurodegenerative disorder that affects nearly one million people in the United States and more than ten million worldwide. It is the second most common neurodegenerative condition after Alzheimer's disease. The hallmark of Parkinson's is the loss of dopamine producing neurons in the brain, which leads to tremors, muscle rigidity, slowed movement, and postural instability. Patients also experience non-motor symptoms such as sleep disturbances, depression, anxiety, and cognitive decline.

The burden of Parkinson's extends far beyond the individual. Families often take on the role of caregivers, adjusting their lives around the physical and emotional needs of a loved one. Daily routines become centered on managing tremors, preventing falls, and providing constant support. The condition is relentless, progressing over time and reshaping households.

THE ENDOCANNABINOID SYSTEM AND PARKINSON'S

The Endocannabinoid System plays a crucial role in motor control, mood regulation, and neuroprotection. CB1 receptors are concentrated in the basal ganglia, the part of the brain that coordinates movement, and CB2 receptors are present in immune cells that regulate inflammation.

In Parkinson's disease, the Endocannabinoid System becomes disrupted. This disruption offers both a challenge and an opportunity. By engaging CB1 receptors, THC helps modulate motor control and reduce tremors. By interacting with CB2 receptors, CBD and other cannabinoids reduce neuroinflammation, protect neurons, and support long term brain health.

Scientists have described Cannabis as a potential neuroprotective agent, not just a symptomatic treatment. In 2014 Dr. Ruth Djaldetti, a neurologist at Tel Aviv University, has said that Cannabis markedly improved motor symptoms such as tremor and rigidity in her Parkinson's patients.

These clinical observations align with what patients have reported for decades: *Cannabis brings balance back to disrupted systems.*

WHAT THE RESEARCH SHOWS

Around the world, researchers have explored the role of Cannabis in Parkinson's disease with encouraging results.

In Israel, a landmark 2014 study at Tel Aviv University followed patients with Parkinson's who used Cannabis. Researchers documented significant improvements in tremor, muscle rigidity, sleep, and pain. Patients also reported reduced falls and improved daily function. Israeli neurologists continue to track Parkinson's patients in national registries, and Cannabis remains a recognized therapy in their system.

In the United Kingdom, the CUPID trial explored whether cannabinoids could slow progression. While the trial faced limitations, it reinforced safety and showed hints of neuroprotection, encouraging further research.

In the United States, the Parkinson's Foundation conducted a survey of more than seven thousand patients and caregivers. Over half reported using Cannabis to manage symptoms, with improvements in sleep, anxiety, pain, and tremor. Despite federal barriers, the survey demonstrated broad acceptance and real world use among American patients.

In Canada, researchers have studied Cannabis for sleep and REM behavior disorder in Parkinson's patients. CBD showed promise in reducing sleep disturbances and improving overall rest. Observational studies also noted improvements in mood and anxiety.

In Europe, German and Italian researchers have conducted trials of Cannabis extracts and nabiximols sprays, showing reductions in spasticity, pain, and tremor intensity. Patients reported greater comfort and smoother daily function.

Animal models provide further evidence. Preclinical research in mice and primates shows that cannabinoids reduce neuroinflammation, protect dopamine producing neurons, and improve motor function. These findings support the idea that Cannabis could slow disease progression, not only treat symptoms.

The consistency across countries is striking. Whether in controlled trials, registries, or surveys, Cannabis improves the quality of life for Parkinson's patients.

PATIENT OUTCOMES AND QUALITY OF LIFE

The effects of Cannabis go beyond clinical charts. Patients with Parkinson's often describe Cannabis as the difference between rigidity and relaxation, between sleepless nights and restorative rest. Tremors that once made eating or writing impossible soften enough for independence to return. Pain from stiffness eases, allowing more freedom of movement.

One patient described Cannabis as the first treatment that allowed him to write his name again after years of tremors. For him, this was not just symptom relief but the restoration of identity and dignity.

Families notice the ripple effect. When tremors lessen and sleep improves, households become calmer. Caregivers feel relief as their loved one is more comfortable and less anxious. Patients regain dignity as they perform daily activities without constant struggle.

Dr. Michael S. Okun, Medical Director of the Parkinson's Foundation, has acknowledged that patients are telling us Cannabis helps with sleep, anxiety, and pain, even if large United States trials have yet to fully confirm the scope. The voices of patients, families, and doctors align in recognizing the benefits.

FORMULATIONS AND APPROACHES

Different Cannabis formulations are used by Parkinson's patients depending on symptoms. Oils and tinctures provide steady relief throughout the day for tremor, stiffness, and anxiety. Vaporization offers rapid control of sudden tremors or muscle spasms. Edibles and gummies provide longer lasting effects that support sleep and nighttime rest. Topicals can reduce localized muscle pain or stiffness. Balanced THC and CBD formulations are often preferred, as THC improves motor control and CBD supports mood and cognition. Terpenes such as linalool and myrcene add relaxation and sleep support, while beta-caryophyllene reinforces anti-inflammatory action.

Patients often work with doctors in Israel, Canada, or Europe to find the right ratio and schedule. In the United States, where structured programs are limited, patients frequently experiment themselves or rely on dispensary guidance.

THE UNITED STATES CHALLENGE VS GLOBAL PROGRESS

The United States has been slow to embrace Cannabis for Parkinson's because of federal restrictions. This has limited funding, delayed large clinical trials, and left patients to rely on anecdotal reports rather than structured guidance.

This is not because of lack of evidence but because of outdated policy and stigma. Patients and caregivers are left navigating a fragmented system while other nations collect structured data and refine best practices.

By contrast, countries like Israel and Canada have integrated Cannabis into national healthcare systems, collecting real world data and guiding physician practice. In Europe, approvals for nabiximols sprays have provided patients with standardized therapies. Australia has added Parkinson's to its rapidly expanding medical Cannabis prescribing system.

The gap between the United States and the rest of the world is clear. While global programs track outcomes and refine best practices, American patients navigate a patchwork system.

POLICY AND ACCESS

Parkinson's disease is recognized as a qualifying condition in many states within the United States, reflecting patient advocacy and need. Yet without federal reform, progress remains fragmented. National organizations such as the Parkinson's Foundation now call for expanded research, better education for doctors, and more consistent access for patients.

Globally, structured programs demonstrate what is possible. Israel and Canada show how national systems can integrate Cannabis into supportive care. The United States has the opportunity to learn from these models and to honor its patients by expanding access and research.

WHY THIS MATTERS

Parkinson's is one of the most feared neurological conditions, not only because of its physical symptoms but because of the way it erodes independence, dignity, and daily joy. Cannabis offers hope where traditional medicines often fall short. It reduces tremors, eases rigidity, restores sleep, calms anxiety, and provides comfort in the face of constant challenges.

This matters because Parkinson's patients and their families have carried an enormous burden with too few options. It matters because Cannabis is not simply easing symptoms but restoring quality of life. It matters because every meal eaten without trembling, every night of restful sleep, and every day lived with more independence is a victory against this disease.

For the United States, closing the research gap is essential. For the world, Cannabis represents compassion in action. For patients and families, it is the difference between enduring and living.

It also matters because Parkinson's patients, like those with MS and cancer, have been some of the earliest advocates in the medical Cannabis movement. Their voices helped legitimize Cannabis as a serious medical therapy and shaped programs that benefit millions today.

Cannabis is not just another treatment for Parkinson's disease. It is a lifeline to dignity, independence, and hope.

12

ARTHRITIS (OSTEOARTHRITIS & RHEUMATOID)

UNDERSTANDING ARTHRITIS

Arthritis is not a single disease but a broad category that includes more than one hundred conditions affecting the joints. The two most common forms are osteoarthritis, a degenerative condition caused by the breakdown of cartilage, and rheumatoid arthritis, an autoimmune disease in which the body's immune system attacks the joints. Together, these conditions affect more than fifty-million adults in the United States and hundreds of millions worldwide.

Osteoarthritis is often described as *"wear and tear"* on the joints. It causes pain, stiffness, swelling, and reduced mobility, most often in the knees, hips, and hands. Rheumatoid arthritis is different. It is systemic, meaning the entire body is involved, and can lead not only to painful inflammation and joint deformities but also to fatigue and other complications throughout the body.

Both conditions impact quality of life, independence, and daily function. Patients live with chronic pain that makes walking, climbing stairs, cooking, or even holding a pen difficult. Families and caregivers carry the burden as they help loved ones manage pain, loss of mobility, and disability.

THE ENDOCANNABINOID SYSTEM AND JOINT HEALTH

The Endocannabinoid System plays a central role in how the body regulates inflammation and pain, both of which are core issues in arthritis. CB1 receptors in the brain and spinal cord regulate the perception of pain, while CB2 receptors in immune cells and joint tissues regulate inflammation and immune response.

In osteoarthritis, cartilage breakdown triggers inflammation that activates nerves inside the joint, causing pain and stiffness. In rheumatoid arthritis, the immune system becomes overactive, releasing inflammatory molecules that attack the joint lining and cause swelling and deformity. Cannabinoids can act on both pathways.

THC engages CB1 receptors to reduce the intensity of pain signals, while CBD and other cannabinoids interact with CB2 receptors to calm inflammation and protect joint tissue. As neurologist and researcher Dr. Ethan Russo has described, Cannabis is a multi-targeted therapy for chronic pain and inflammation, which makes it uniquely suited to arthritis.

RESEARCH EVIDENCE AROUND THE WORLD

The scientific evidence for Cannabis in arthritis is steadily growing, and international studies provide strong insights.

Canada: *Clinical trials of nabiximols, a THC and CBD oral spray, showed reduced pain and improved sleep in rheumatoid arthritis patients, along with less morning stiffness and better mobility.*

United Kingdom: *Research in inflammatory joint models confirmed both anti-inflammatory and pain relieving effects of cannabinoids.*

Israel: *Registry data covering thousands of arthritis patients shows sustained reductions in pain, improvements in sleep, and reduced reliance on opioids and non-steroidal anti-inflammatories.*

United States: *Surveys from the Arthritis Foundation reveal that more than half of arthritis patients report using Cannabis or CBD. The majority describe meaningful improvements in pain, sleep, and anxiety. Federal restrictions, however, have limited large-scale US clinical trials.*

Europe: *Studies in Germany, Italy, and the Netherlands show that Cannabis extracts and CBD oils reduce pain and improve daily function, particularly when combined with conventional care.*

Australia: *Prescription data confirms arthritis as one of the top conditions for which Cannabis is prescribed, with oils and capsules commonly used to reduce pain and stiffness.*

Across continents, the consensus is clear. Cannabis reduces pain, improves sleep, and enhances quality of life for arthritis patients.

SYMPTOM RELIEF IN DAILY LIFE

Patients consistently report that Cannabis eases joint pain at rest and during movement, reduces stiffness in the mornings, calms swelling, and restores sleep. CBD-rich formulations are especially effective for inflammation and tenderness, while balanced THC and CBD products are valued for sleep support and mood stability.

Relief from constant pain also improves mental health. Patients often describe reduced anxiety, less irritability, and more emotional resilience. For many, Cannabis makes the difference between a day defined by pain and a day lived with dignity and participation.

PATIENT OUTCOMES AND FAMILY PERSPECTIVES

Real-world experiences echo the science. Arthritis patients frequently reduce or discontinue opioids, anti-inflammatories, and sleep medications when Cannabis becomes part of their care. Families describe seeing loved ones return to gardening, walking, or cooking again.

One patient said Cannabis was the first thing that allowed her to spend time in the garden without crippling pain. For her, Cannabis was not simply about symptom relief, it was about reclaiming joy and identity. Caregivers also report less stress as their loved ones regain independence.

Dr. Mary Ann Fitzcharles, a rheumatologist at McGill University, has observed that patients with chronic arthritis pain often find Cannabis to be one of the few treatments that restores function with fewer disabling side effects.

FORMULATIONS AND APPROACHES

Cannabis offers multiple delivery methods suited to arthritis care. Oils and tinctures provide steady relief throughout the day. Edibles and capsules offer longer-lasting effects, especially for sleep. Topical creams and balms applied directly to joints provide localized anti-inflammatory relief, while vaporization can bring rapid relief during acute flare-ups.

Balanced THC and CBD oils are often effective for both osteoarthritis and rheumatoid arthritis. Terpenes add another dimension with beta-caryophyllene supporting inflammation control, linalool calming anxiety, and myrcene promoting restful sleep. Many patients combine systemic relief with topical applications to manage daily pain and sudden spikes.

THE UNITED STATES CHALLENGE VS GLOBAL PROGRESS

While patients in Israel, Canada, and Europe benefit from structured programs and physician-guided dosing, the United States still lags behind. Federal restrictions have slowed clinical trials and left most patients to rely on anecdotal evidence or state level programs.

This gap is not caused by lack of science but by outdated policy. Arthritis affects tens of millions of Americans, yet national funding, clinical training, and insurance coverage remain limited. Despite this, arthritis is recognized as a qualifying condition in many state programs, and millions of patients are already turning to Cannabis for relief.

The Arthritis Foundation itself, one of the largest advocacy groups, has called for more research and for Cannabis to be considered a serious part of comprehensive arthritis care.

POLICY AND ACCESS

Globally, Cannabis is steadily becoming integrated into arthritis care. Canada, Israel, and much of Europe lead with structured national systems, while Australia continues to expand prescribing. In the United States, advocacy organizations and patient groups are pushing for federal reform, insurance coverage, and better physician education.

WHY THIS MATTERS

Arthritis is one of the most common and disabling conditions in the world. It steals mobility, independence, and quality of life. It places emotional and financial burdens on families and costs societies billions in healthcare expenses and lost productivity.

Cannabis changes this story. It reduces pain, restores sleep, and improves mobility. It gives patients dignity and independence. It gives caregivers relief and families hope.

This matters because arthritis patients represent one of the largest groups in the medical Cannabis movement. Their stories and advocacy have reshaped public opinion and continue to drive reform at every level. It matters because Cannabis is one of the few treatments that addresses pain, inflammation, sleep, and mood together. Every step taken without pain, every night of restorative sleep, and every day lived with less stiffness is a victory.

For the United States, embracing Cannabis for arthritis is a chance to align with global progress and honor the millions who already use it successfully.

For the world, it is an opportunity to provide compassionate, effective care for one of the most widespread conditions of our time.

Cannabis is not just an alternative therapy for arthritis. It is an essential tool for restoring lives, families, and communities.

13

CROHN'S DISEASE & IBS

UNDERSTANDING CROHN'S DISEASE AND IBS

Crohn's disease is a chronic inflammatory bowel condition that can affect any part of the digestive tract, most often the small intestine and colon. It causes abdominal pain, severe diarrhea, weight loss, fatigue, and malnutrition. The condition is unpredictable, marked by flare-ups and remissions that disrupt daily life. In the United States, more than three million people live with inflammatory bowel diseases such as Crohn's and ulcerative colitis. Globally, rates are rising, particularly in industrialized nations.

Irritable bowel syndrome *(IBS)* is different but equally disruptive. It affects up to 15 percent of the United States population and is characterized by abdominal pain, bloating, and alternating diarrhea or constipation. Unlike Crohn's, IBS does not involve structural damage or inflammation but is linked to disordered gut brain communication. Both conditions diminish quality of life, limit social participation, and create heavy emotional burdens for patients and families.

THE ENDOCANNABINOID SYSTEM AND DIGESTIVE HEALTH

The digestive system contains one of the body's highest concentrations of endocannabinoid receptors. CB1 receptors in the gut regulate motility, pain perception, and secretion, while CB2 receptors in immune cells control inflammation and immune activity.

In Crohn's disease, an overactive immune response damages intestinal tissue and drives inflammation. In IBS, disrupted communication between the brain and gut leads to spasms, pain, and irregular bowel movements. Cannabinoids influence both pathways. THC reduces motility and spasms, easing cramping and diarrhea. CBD calms immune activity, lowers inflammation, and restores balance.

Dr. Mauro Maccarrone, an Italian researcher on the Endocannabinoid System, has described cannabinoids as *"critical regulators of intestinal homeostasis,"* emphasizing their ability to restore equilibrium in disrupted gut systems.

RESEARCH EVIDENCE AROUND THE WORLD

In Israel, Dr. Timna Naftali conducted a landmark study in 2013 showing that most Crohn's patients who used Cannabis reported significant reductions in pain and diarrhea, with nearly half achieving full remission. Later follow-ups documented improved appetite and weight gain. Israel's national program continues to support patients with Crohn's and ulcerative colitis.

In Canada, observational studies show that patients with Crohn's and IBS experience fewer flare-ups, less abdominal pain, and reduced reliance on corticosteroids when using Cannabis. Surveys confirm high satisfaction among patients who incorporate Cannabis into their care.

In the United States, research at the University of Chicago found that Crohn's patients reported improved quality of life and reduced dependence on narcotic medications after using Cannabis. Surveys from the Crohn's and Colitis Foundation indicate that one in four patients has tried Cannabis, with many noting improvements in pain, appetite, and sleep.

Across Europe, Dutch researchers found reductions in inflammation markers and improvements in daily function. German physicians routinely prescribe Cannabis for inflammatory bowel disease through national health programs. In Australia, prescription data shows a steady increase in Cannabis use for gastrointestinal disorders, with patients reporting relief from nausea, improved appetite, and more predictable bowel habits.

The findings from country to country are remarkably consistent. Cannabis improves symptoms and restores quality of life, often when standard treatments fall short.

HOW CANNABIS HELPS WITH CORE SYMPTOMS

Cannabis addresses multiple symptoms of Crohn's disease and IBS at once. Patients often describe less abdominal cramping and reduced spasms as THC and CBD calm overactive nerves in the intestines. THC slows bowel motility, easing frequent or urgent trips to the bathroom. CBD reduces immune system overactivity in Crohn's, which lowers inflammation and limits tissue damage.

Beyond the gut itself, Cannabis restores appetite and supports healthy weight in patients struggling with malnutrition. It also improves sleep and reduces the anxiety that accompanies chronic illness. These combined effects help patients regain confidence in their bodies and return to a more normal daily rhythm.

PATIENT OUTCOMES AND QUALITY OF LIFE

Registry data and surveys confirm what patients and families describe in their own words. Many reduce or stop using steroids, opioids, and anti-diarrheal medications when they begin Cannabis therapy. This not only lowers the risk of side effects but also improves long term stability.

Families report that stress decreases as flare-ups become less frequent and less severe. A patient in Israel described Cannabis as *"the first treatment that let me eat without fear."* A United States patient said she was able to attend her daughter's graduation without worrying about bathroom access. Another explained that Cannabis finally allowed him to sit through family dinners without constant pain.

These stories highlight what the data makes clear: *Cannabis is more than symptom relief.*

It restores dignity and allows people to rejoin the fabric of daily life.

FORMULATIONS AND APPROACHES

Patients with Crohn's and IBS use a variety of formulations depending on symptoms and lifestyle. Oils and tinctures provide steady control for inflammation and pain, while capsules deliver consistent daily dosing. Vaporization offers rapid relief for sudden cramps or spasms, and edibles provide longer lasting support through the night.

Balanced THC and CBD formulations are especially effective for Crohn's disease, since they target both inflammation and intestinal spasms. Patients with IBS often prefer CBD forward products that ease cramping and anxiety without producing strong intoxication. Terpenes add another layer of support, with beta-caryophyllene reducing inflammation, limonene lifting mood, and linalool calming stress.

THE UNITED STATES CHALLENGE VS GLOBAL PROGRESS

While many US states recognize Crohn's disease as a qualifying condition for medical Cannabis, federal restrictions continue to limit research and physician guidance. Patients often rely on dispensaries or self directed experimentation rather than structured medical oversight.

By contrast, Israel and Canada collect comprehensive patient data through national programs, allowing doctors to refine dosing strategies and track long term outcomes. Europe and Australia have also integrated Cannabis into structured gastrointestinal care.

The difference is striking: *while American patients face uncertainty, patients abroad benefit from guided treatment and real world evidence.*

POLICY AND ACCESS

In the United States, advocacy groups such as the Crohn's and Colitis Foundation have called for more research, education, and physician training on Cannabis. Globally, governments and health systems are beginning to view Cannabis as a legitimate tool in gastrointestinal care. Policies are gradually shifting toward wider access and integration, reflecting both patient demand and scientific evidence.

WHY THIS MATTERS

Crohn's disease and IBS strip away a sense of normalcy. They dictate daily routines, create social anxiety, and erode quality of life. For patients, the battle is not just physical but emotional and social.

Cannabis changes that story. It calms spasms, restores appetite, reduces inflammation, and improves sleep. It lowers dependence on steroids and narcotics, offering safer long term care. Most importantly, it gives patients back confidence in their bodies and dignity in their lives.

This matters because millions of people live with these conditions in silence, often dismissed or told their suffering was imagined. Cannabis validates their experiences and provides tangible relief. For the United States, embracing Cannabis means catching up to global progress and honoring the voices of patients who already know its benefits. For the world, it means delivering compassionate, comprehensive care to millions who need it.

Cannabis is not just symptom relief for Crohn's disease and IBS. It is a pathway back to dignity, independence, and quality of life.

14

GLAUCOMA

UNDERSTANDING GLAUCOMA

Glaucoma is one of the leading causes of irreversible blindness worldwide. It affects more than three million people in the United States and an estimated seventy-six million globally. The disease is defined by progressive damage to the optic nerve, often linked to elevated intraocular pressure *(IOP)*. Over time, untreated glaucoma narrows vision from the periphery inward until central sight is lost.

The condition is often called the silent thief of sight because it progresses slowly and without early warning signs. Many people are unaware they have glaucoma until vision loss is already advanced. Standard treatments include prescription eye drops, oral medications, laser therapies, and surgery. These therapies aim to reduce intraocular pressure, but they are not always effective or well tolerated. For this reason, Cannabis has become an area of interest for both patients and researchers.

THE ENDOCANNABINOID SYSTEM AND EYE HEALTH

The eye contains a high density of endocannabinoid receptors, especially in the ciliary body, retina, and trabecular meshwork, which regulates fluid drainage and intraocular pressure. CB1 receptors influence aqueous humor production and drainage, directly affecting eye pressure. CB2 receptors are found in retinal tissue and immune cells, where they may reduce oxidative stress and inflammation that damage the optic nerve.

Cannabinoids such as THC and CBD interact with these receptors in ways that influence intraocular pressure, blood flow to the optic nerve, and retinal health. The eye also produces its own endocannabinoids, which help regulate pressure and protect nerve tissue.

Dr. Gary Novack, a California ophthalmologist and researcher, has noted that cannabinoids exert real effects on intraocular pressure and deserve careful scientific study.

RESEARCH EVIDENCE AROUND THE WORLD

In the United States, pioneering studies at UCLA in the 1970s demonstrated that smoking Cannabis reduced intraocular pressure by about twenty-five percent in glaucoma patients. However, the effects lasted only three to four hours, making continuous relief difficult.

In Israel, researchers have focused on oral and sublingual cannabinoid formulations. THC and synthetic analogues lowered intraocular pressure, while CBD produced mixed results depending on dosage. Israeli teams are also exploring whether cannabinoids protect retinal cells from damage.

In Canada, observational reports from medical Cannabis patients confirm reductions in eye pressure, along with better sleep and improved quality of life. Canadian ophthalmologists emphasize the importance of new delivery methods to make Cannabis more practical as a therapy.

In Europe, studies in the United Kingdom and Germany showed that THC lowered eye pressure and improved ocular blood flow, which may help protect the optic nerve. Trials of nabiximols sprays and oral extracts produced encouraging results, though effectiveness varied by dose and ratio.

Animal studies also show that cannabinoids protect retinal ganglion cells, reduce oxidative stress, and support blood flow to the optic nerve, suggesting benefits beyond pressure reduction.

The evidence is consistent across regions. Cannabinoids lower intraocular pressure, but they may also protect vision in ways that standard drugs cannot.

HOW CANNABIS HELPS WITH CORE SYMPTOMS

Cannabis provides support for glaucoma patients in several ways. THC reduces intraocular pressure by lowering aqueous humor production and improving fluid drainage. Cannabinoids protect retinal cells and the optic nerve from oxidative stress and inflammation. Blood flow to the optic nerve improves, which is critical for preserving sight.

Many patients also experience relief from ocular pain, headaches, or eye strain. Better comfort translates into deeper and more restorative sleep.

WHY CANNABIS CAUSES RED EYES

One of the most visible effects of Cannabis use is redness of the eyes, a detail often misunderstood and stigmatized. This effect is not a sign of impairment or poor health, but rather a direct reflection of the plant's therapeutic action. THC lowers blood pressure and dilates blood vessels, including the tiny capillaries in the eyes. As these vessels widen, blood flow increases and intraocular pressure drops, providing relief for glaucoma patients. The same process that eases pressure also makes the vessels more visible, giving the eyes a temporary red or *"bloodshot"* appearance. Far from being a symbol of misuse, it is evidence of the body's vascular response working exactly as intended.

PATIENT OUTCOMES AND QUALITY OF LIFE

Patients often describe Cannabis as the first therapy that provided noticeable relief from eye pressure and discomfort. In surveys by the American Glaucoma Society, many reported turning to Cannabis when prescription medications caused intolerable side effects or failed to control pressure.

One patient explained, *"I can feel the difference within minutes, as if a weight has been lifted off my eyes."* Another described finally being able to read without constant blur or ache. A grandmother shared that Cannabis allowed her to clearly recognize her grandchild's face for the first time in months. Families also report less stress when loved ones find comfort and more consistent sleep.

FORMULATIONS AND APPROACHES

Patients with glaucoma use Cannabis in several forms depending on their needs. Inhalation through smoking or vaporization provides the fastest reduction in eye pressure, though the effect is brief. Oils, tinctures, and capsules offer steadier dosing and longer duration of relief, though capsules may take longer to act.

Topical eye drops containing cannabinoids are under active development, but absorption challenges remain. Balanced THC and CBD formulations may provide both pressure reduction and neuroprotection. Terpenes such as limonene and pinene add potential support by improving circulation and reducing oxidative stress.

Looking ahead, the future of glaucoma care will likely depend on improved cannabinoid delivery systems, particularly eye drops or targeted therapies that extend relief without producing unwanted psychoactive effects.

THE UNITED STATES CHALLENGE VS GLOBAL PROGRESS

In the United States, glaucoma is one of the most recognized qualifying conditions in medical Cannabis programs. Patients in dozens of states legally use Cannabis to manage symptoms. Yet federal restrictions continue to block large-scale trials and slow the development of advanced cannabinoid therapies.

By contrast, Israel and parts of Europe are actively developing cannabinoid-based eye drops and oral formulations through government-backed programs. Canada includes glaucoma in its national framework, collecting structured data to guide practice. Australia continues to expand medical Cannabis prescribing, with glaucoma listed among approved conditions.

The United States risks falling behind by failing to transform Cannabis from an informal option into a validated medical treatment.

POLICY AND ACCESS

The American Glaucoma Society acknowledges the real effects of Cannabis but calls for more research to refine delivery and dosing. Advocacy groups argue that patients should not be denied access to a therapy that provides relief, even if imperfect. Globally, governments are moving toward integrating Cannabis into ocular care, with Israel, Canada, Europe, and Australia leading the way.

WHY THIS MATTERS

Glaucoma is irreversible. Once vision is lost, it cannot be regained. Every therapy that slows progression or preserves sight is critical. Cannabis lowers intraocular pressure but also offers neuroprotection and improvements in quality of life beyond what standard medications provide.

This matters because millions worldwide face blindness despite current treatments. It matters because Cannabis is safe, effective, and empowers patients to participate actively in their care. It matters because preserving vision is preserving independence, dignity, and life itself.

It also matters because glaucoma patients were among the earliest advocates for medical Cannabis in the 1970s. Their voices helped launch the modern movement and pushed Cannabis into mainstream medical debate decades before legalization.

For the United States, embracing Cannabis research in glaucoma means catching up to global leaders and providing patients with new hope. For the world, it means ensuring that the silent thief of sight is met with every tool available.

Cannabis is not just relief for glaucoma. It is a chance to preserve the gift of sight and to honor the patients who helped shape the medical Cannabis movement.

15

MENTAL HEALTH CONDITIONS (ANXIETY, DEPRESSION & PTSD)

UNDERSTANDING MENTAL HEALTH CONDITIONS

Mental health disorders are among the most widespread and disabling conditions in the world. In the United States, nearly one in five adults lives with a diagnosable disorder. Anxiety affects more than forty-million Americans, major depression remains a leading cause of disability, and post-traumatic stress disorder disrupts the lives of millions globally.

The cost is measured not only in statistics but in human suffering. Families are torn apart, lives are cut short by suicide, and patients often endure years of trial and error with prescription medications. Cannabis has emerged as a natural option that addresses mood, stress, sleep, and resilience in ways that feel more holistic and accessible.

THE ENDOCANNABINOID SYSTEM AND MENTAL HEALTH

The Endocannabinoid System regulates mood, fear responses, memory, and recovery from stress. CB1 receptors dominate in brain regions that govern emotion and memory, while CB2 receptors influence inflammation, which is increasingly tied to depression and anxiety.

THC engages CB1 receptors to quiet hyperactive fear circuits. CBD modulates serotonin and stress pathways. Together, these cannabinoids restore balance to disrupted networks. Dr. Raphael Mechoulam once described the ECS as a bridge between body and mind, explaining why Cannabis influences both physical and emotional health.

RESEARCH EVIDENCE AROUND THE WORLD

A 2021 survey from Johns Hopkins University followed more than three thousand PTSD patients and found Cannabis reduced the severity of symptoms, nightmares, and insomnia. Veterans in Colorado showed similar improvements, including better sleep and fewer intrusive memories.

For anxiety, Yale University and University College London confirmed that CBD reduces measurable anxiety during stressful public speaking tests. In Canada, researchers at McGill University reported that Cannabis reduced both anxiety and depression while also improving sleep quality. Registry studies from multiple countries show patients often reduce reliance on antidepressants and experience fewer hospitalizations when Cannabis is integrated into care.

In Israel, the University of Haifa demonstrated that Cannabis calmed fear circuits and reduced trauma-related behaviors. Tel Aviv University showed that THC helped extinguish traumatic memories. In Australia, the University of Sydney's Lambert Initiative found Cannabis prescriptions improved sleep and stability for PTSD and anxiety patients. Across Europe, CBD-rich formulations supported mood regulation and reduced generalized anxiety.

ANXIETY DISORDERS

Anxiety disorders are defined by excessive worry, panic, and physical symptoms that disrupt daily life. THC reduces overactivity in the amygdala, while CBD regulates serotonin and stress responses. Patients describe Cannabis as a way to breathe again and regain calm in overwhelming situations.

DEPRESSION

Depression brings persistent sadness, loss of interest, changes in appetite and sleep, and difficulty concentrating. Antidepressants often take weeks to work and cause side effects that patients struggle to tolerate. Cannabis offers another path.

THC elevates mood by influencing dopamine pathways, while CBD promotes neurogenesis in the hippocampus, a brain region often damaged in depression. Studies from McGill University found that Cannabis patients experienced reduced depressive symptoms and improved quality of life. Patients often describe Cannabis as reconnecting them with joy, motivation, and simple pleasures that once felt unreachable.

POST-TRAUMATIC STRESS DISORDER

PTSD develops after trauma and is defined by flashbacks, nightmares, hypervigilance, and emotional numbness. Cannabis has shown remarkable promise in this area. Johns Hopkins confirmed reductions in PTSD symptoms and improvements in sleep.

In Israel, researchers demonstrated that THC helps the brain extinguish intrusive memories, while CBD reduces anxiety and calms the nervous system. Veterans in the United States frequently report that Cannabis allows them to rest, reconnect with family, and manage stress. Many credit Cannabis with preventing suicidal thoughts when every other therapy failed.

HOW CANNABIS HELPS WITH CORE SYMPTOMS

Cannabis addresses several aspects of mental health at once. For anxiety, it calms the amygdala and restores a sense of safety. For depression, it elevates mood and supports the growth of new brain cells. For PTSD, it reduces nightmares, eases hypervigilance, and helps extinguish traumatic associations. Cannabis also improves sleep, shortens the time to fall asleep, and deepens rest. By lowering cortisol and calming overactive circuits, it strengthens resilience against stress.

PATIENT OUTCOMES AND QUALITY OF LIFE

Patients consistently report life-changing improvements. Those with anxiety feel calm enough to rejoin social life. Those with depression regain motivation for daily tasks. Veterans with PTSD describe sleeping peacefully for the first time in years.

Families notice the difference. Many say Cannabis brought back the person they thought they had lost. These moments of restoration ripple across households, lifting caregivers and renewing hope.

FORMULATIONS AND APPROACHES

Patients use Cannabis in many forms depending on their needs. CBD oils provide calm without intoxication. Balanced THC and CBD oils support mood and sleep. Vaporization brings rapid relief during panic attacks, while edibles provide stability through the night. Capsules ensure consistent dosing. Terpenes such as linalool, myrcene, and limonene fine-tune the effects, supporting relaxation, rest, or uplifted mood.

THE UNITED STATES CHALLENGE VS GLOBAL PROGRESS

In the United States, mental health conditions are not always recognized as qualifying conditions despite overwhelming patient demand. Federal restrictions limit trials and physician guidance, leaving many patients to self-navigate.

By contrast, Israel, Canada, and Australia integrate Cannabis into structured psychiatric care. Europe has begun approving CBD based medicines for anxiety and sleep. The United States risks falling behind in an area where patients urgently seek relief.

POLICY AND ACCESS

Advocacy groups including the American Legion, veterans' organizations, and mental health nonprofits continue to call for broader access. Globally, governments are investing in trials and integrating Cannabis into mental health care. The momentum is clear, Cannabis is increasingly recognized as a tool for healing invisible wounds and preventing suicide.

WHY THIS MATTERS

Mental health defines how people think, feel, and connect with others. Disorders such as anxiety, depression, and PTSD disrupt every aspect of life and heighten the risk of suicide.

Cannabis changes this story. It restores sleep, lifts mood, calms fear, and reconnects people with their loved ones. It provides veterans with peace, children with resilience, and families with hope.

For the United States, embracing Cannabis for mental health means preventing suicides, restoring families, and honoring survivors. For the world, it means recognizing Cannabis as a central tool in the future of psychiatry.

Cannabis is not just symptom relief for anxiety, depression, and PTSD. It is a pathway to resilience, recovery, and hope.

16

MIGRAINES & HEADACHES

UNDERSTANDING MIGRAINES AND HEADACHES

Migraines are far more than ordinary headaches. They are a complex neurological disorder that affects more than thirty-nine million people in the United States and more than one billion worldwide. This makes migraines one of the most common and disabling conditions on earth.

Migraine attacks often bring severe throbbing pain, usually on one side of the head, and are frequently accompanied by nausea, vomiting, and heightened sensitivity to light and sound. These episodes can last from hours to several days, forcing patients into dark, quiet rooms and disrupting work, family life, and social activities.

Headaches more broadly, including tension headaches and cluster headaches, also take a heavy toll. Cluster headaches are sometimes called *"suicide headaches"* because of their intensity. Standard treatments such as triptans, anti-inflammatories, anti-seizure medications, and preventive drugs can help some patients, but many find them ineffective or difficult to tolerate. This is where Cannabis has drawn increasing attention as an alternative or complementary option.

THE ENDOCANNABINOID SYSTEM AND HEAD PAIN

The Endocannabinoid System plays a central role in regulating pain, blood vessel tone, and neurological signaling. CB1 receptors located in the brainstem, cortex, and trigeminal nerve pathways influence how pain is transmitted and perceived. CB2 receptors regulate inflammation, which can worsen migraine activity.

THC interacts with CB1 receptors to reduce pain signaling, while CBD calms inflammation and supports serotonin pathways that are also involved in migraine attacks. Some researchers have proposed that a condition known as clinical endocannabinoid deficiency helps explain why certain people are more prone to migraines. In 2004, Dr. Ethan Russo suggested that low endocannabinoid activity may underlie migraines, fibromyalgia, and irritable bowel syndrome, all of which respond to Cannabis. This theory, first introduced in Chapter 3, reinforces why Cannabis is uniquely effective for migraine sufferers.

RESEARCH EVIDENCE AROUND THE WORLD

Research from multiple countries has produced consistent and encouraging results.

In the United States, a 2019 study from the University of Colorado found that medical Cannabis use reduced the average number of monthly migraine attacks by more than half, from around ten per month to about four. Patients also reported shorter migraine duration and less reliance on prescription medication.

Italian researchers in 2018 studied patients with chronic migraines who used Cannabis oil extracts. They documented meaningful reductions in pain intensity and frequency, as well as improvements in sleep and overall quality of life.

Observational data from Israel's medical Cannabis program further confirmed reductions in headache frequency and severity, with many patients reporting relief where conventional therapies had failed. Canadian registry studies revealed similar outcomes, showing fewer migraine days, reduced use of opioids and triptans, and better rest.

A 2020 global review concluded that Cannabis and cannabinoids consistently reduce migraine pain, frequency, and medication reliance, though additional controlled trials are still needed to strengthen the evidence base.

HOW CANNABIS HELPS WITH SYMPTOMS

Patients describe improvements across several domains. The frequency of attacks often decreases, and when migraines do occur, they are less intense. Nausea and vomiting, among the most disabling features of migraines, are reduced. Patients also report fewer visual disturbances and less sensitivity to sound or light during episodes. Better sleep is another consistent benefit, and since poor sleep is itself a migraine trigger, this creates a reinforcing cycle of stability.

Perhaps most importantly, patients frequently reduce or even eliminate their dependence on opioids, triptans, or anti-nausea drugs once Cannabis is incorporated into care.

PATIENT OUTCOMES AND QUALITY OF LIFE

The lived experiences behind the numbers highlight Cannabis's true value. In the Colorado study, one patient explained that for the first time in years they could go days without debilitating pain. Italian patients described Cannabis as giving them back their nights, allowing them to rest instead of enduring hours of agony.

Others speak of restored participation in daily life, attending a child's school play without fear of retreating to a dark room, or sharing a family dinner without the constant threat of an attack. Families notice the difference too, as stress and disruption lessen when migraines are better controlled.

FORMULATIONS AND APPROACHES

Patients use Cannabis in different ways depending on their needs. Inhalation through vaporization provides rapid relief during acute migraine attacks, though the effects are shorter lived. Oils and tinctures are often taken preventively to reduce the frequency of migraines. Capsules provide consistent daily dosing for those with chronic patterns, while edibles extend relief through the night. Topical applications can help with tension headaches when applied to the temples, forehead, or neck.

Balanced formulations containing both THC and CBD are commonly favored, as they combine rapid pain relief with anti-inflammatory and calming properties. Terpenes contribute additional layers of effect. Limonene and pinene are associated with mental clarity and uplifted mood, while linalool and myrcene support relaxation and rest.

THE UNITED STATES CHALLENGE VS GLOBAL PROGRESS

In the United States, migraines are not always recognized as a qualifying condition in medical Cannabis programs, forcing patients to seek treatment under broader categories such as chronic pain. Federal restrictions also limit clinical trials and physician education. Despite these obstacles, migraines remain one of the most common reasons patients self medicate with Cannabis, underscoring the gap between patient demand and formal recognition.

Globally, countries like Italy, Israel, and Canada openly recognize migraines and headaches as legitimate reasons for Cannabis prescriptions. These nations integrate treatment into neurology clinics, track patient outcomes, and refine dosing protocols, giving patients structured guidance that many Americans still lack.

POLICY AND ACCESS

Advocacy groups in the United States continue to push for migraines and headaches to be explicitly included in state medical Cannabis programs. Internationally, policymakers are expanding access as evidence grows. The World Health Organization has acknowledged the global burden of migraines, further pressing for innovation and compassionate care.

WHY THIS MATTERS

Migraines and headaches are among the most common medical conditions in the world, yet they remain under treated for millions. They strip away productivity, limit family participation, and create constant fear of the next attack.

Cannabis offers a new story. It reduces the frequency and severity of attacks, alleviates nausea and sensory disruption, restores sleep, and gives patients back control over their lives. For families, it means less stress and more shared experiences. For society, it represents a therapy that can reduce medication reliance and restore quality of life for countless people.

This matters because migraines affect more than a billion people worldwide. Every pain free day, every restful night, and every moment of regained normalcy is a victory. For the United States, expanding Cannabis for migraines means catching up to nations already leading the way. For the world, it means providing compassionate and effective care for one of humanity's most widespread and disabling disorders.

Cannabis is not just an alternative for migraines and headaches. It is a pathway to freedom from suffering, dignity restored, and life reclaimed.

17

DIABETES & METABOLIC DISORDERS

UNDERSTANDING DIABETES AND METABOLIC HEALTH

Diabetes is one of the defining health challenges of our time, in the United States and around the world. Type one diabetes requires insulin from outside the body. Type two diabetes is driven by insulin resistance and loss of beta cell function over time. Metabolic disorders such as metabolic syndrome and fatty liver often travel with diabetes, magnifying the risks to the heart, kidneys, eyes, and nerves.

Patients live with glucose swings, fatigue, neuropathic pain, and constant stress. Standard care helps many, yet large numbers still struggle with daily control, restful sleep, and quality of life.

This is where Cannabis based care has begun to play a meaningful role: *easing pain, improving rest, supporting appetite regulation, and reshaping the biology of metabolism through its influence on the Endocannabinoid System.*

THE ENDOCANNABINOID SYSTEM AND METABOLISM

The Endocannabinoid System is a master regulator of energy balance. CB1 receptors in the brain, liver, and fat tissue influence hunger signals, insulin sensitivity, and the way the body stores or burns fuel. CB2 receptors in immune cells modulate inflammation, which is directly linked to insulin resistance.

Modern reviews show that overactive CB1 activity in the liver promotes fatty acid synthesis and contributes to diet driven obesity. Rebalancing this system improves glucose handling and lipid metabolism. These insights highlight why cannabinoids are being studied not only for symptom relief, but for their potential role in improving metabolic health at its root.

WHAT THE DATA SHOWS IN THE UNITED STATES

Large US population studies have reported a consistent signal. Adults who reported current Cannabis use had lower fasting insulin, lower levels of insulin resistance, and smaller waist circumference compared with non-users.

Cannabis also helps with one of the most stubborn complications of diabetes: *painful peripheral neuropathy.*

A placebo controlled trial at the University of California San Diego demonstrated that inhaled Cannabis reduced neuropathic pain in a dose dependent fashion for patients with treatment resistant diabetic neuropathy. This provided controlled human evidence to back what many patients had long reported.

TARGETED CANNABINOIDS FOR GLUCOSE CONTROL

Beyond whole-plant medicine, researchers are studying specific cannabinoids for direct metabolic benefits. In a landmark randomized, double blind study in people with type two diabetes, the rare cannabinoid THCV improved fasting glucose and measures of beta cell function without intoxication. This trial suggests that cannabinoid profiles can be fine-tuned for glycemic control as well as for symptom relief.

LIVER HEALTH AND METABOLIC SYNDROME

Metabolic dysfunction often appears in the liver as fatty liver disease. Several large US database analyses found that current Cannabis users had a lower prevalence of non-alcoholic fatty liver disease, even after adjusting for metabolic risk factors. While observational data cannot prove causation, the consistent association is notable and aligns with the biology of endocannabinoid signaling in the liver.

INTERNATIONAL EVIDENCE

International data strengthens the case. Canadian registries tracking thousands of medical Cannabis patients consistently show improvements in pain, sleep, and daily function for people living with diabetes and metabolic disorders. In Israel, clinical programs report neuropathy relief and better sleep as common outcomes. European research adds mechanistic insight, highlighting cannabinoid roles in reducing inflammation, oxidative stress, and microvascular damage. In Australia, university groups report that Cannabis prescriptions improve rest and stress management, indirectly supporting glucose stability and overall health.

HOW CANNABIS HELPS DAY TO DAY

For many patients, Cannabis provides tangible daily benefits. Neuropathic pain becomes less overwhelming, allowing longer walks and more restful nights. Sleep deepens and becomes steadier, an essential factor since poor sleep worsens insulin resistance. Stress levels fall, moods stabilize, and glucose patterns become less erratic. Appetite regulation also improves, with fewer late-night binges and more consistent mealtimes. Inflammation is calmed through gentle modulation of immune pathways that interact with insulin signaling.

FORMULATIONS AND APPROACHES

Cannabis can be tailored to individual needs. Oils and tinctures provide steady daytime relief for stress, sleep, and neuropathic discomfort. Capsules offer consistency for those who prefer a set routine. Vaporization delivers rapid relief during flare-ups of neuropathic pain, while edibles extend support through the night. Topical creams can be applied to painful feet or lower legs, easing discomfort without affecting cognition.

Minor cannabinoids add another layer of precision. THCV shows promise for glycemic control, while CBD balanced with small amounts of THC can reduce pain and improve sleep without impairing daily function.

WHY THE UNITED STATES NEEDS TO LEAD

The United States carries one of the heaviest burdens of type two diabetes and metabolic disease, yet federal research infrastructure has lagged. Schedule I restrictions have created layers of approvals and sourcing barriers that slowed randomized trials and product standardization, even as millions of patients sought relief.

National Academies reviews have urged a more modern public health approach to Cannabis policy. Media coverage has tracked proposals to ease research restrictions and align federal law with state realities. Every step toward research access brings patients closer to guidance on dosing, delivery methods, and long term outcomes.

WHY THIS MATTERS

Diabetes and metabolic disorders shape how people live every day. They influence energy, sleep, pain, and long term health risks. Cannabis is not a cure, but evidence shows clear reasons to include it in comprehensive care. It reduces neuropathic pain, improves sleep, moderates stress, and interacts with metabolic biology in ways that support healthier glucose control and liver function.

The evidence from US cohorts, targeted cannabinoid trials, and global clinical programs all point in the same direction: *compassionate, structured Cannabis care can improve life for people with diabetes.*

For patients and families, this means fewer nights of burning pain, more mornings with energy, and steadier days. For clinicians, it adds another evidence-backed tool to complement nutrition, physical activity, medications, and monitoring. For policymakers, it is a call to align science with patient needs.

Cannabis is not a cure-all, but it is a practical instrument in the orchestra of diabetes care. It supports comfort, rest, and resilience while working in harmony with the biology of metabolic health. That is worth embracing, studying, and delivering with quality and compassion.

Cannabis is not a cure-all, but it is a practical instrument in the orchestra of diabetes care.

18

AUTISM SPECTRUM & ASPERGER'S

UNDERSTANDING AUTISM SPECTRUM

Autism spectrum disorder is a neurodevelopmental condition that affects communication, social interaction, sensory processing, and behavior. It is called a spectrum because strengths and challenges vary widely from person to person. In the United States, the number of children identified on the spectrum has risen in recent years as awareness and screening have improved. Families often navigate complex care that includes behavioral therapies, school supports, and medications prescribed off label for irritability or sleep.

When these conventional approaches are not enough, many parents and clinicians explore Cannabis based therapies. Across the world, researchers have examined how cannabinoids may support regulation of behavior, improve rest, and reduce self-harm or aggressive outbursts. Emerging evidence shows that Cannabis can also enhance social responsiveness and stabilize daily routines.

THE ENDOCANNABINOID SYSTEM AND NEURODEVELOPMENT

The Endocannabinoid System plays a central role in neurodevelopment and ongoing brain function. CB1 receptors are concentrated in the cortex, hippocampus, amygdala, and basal ganglia, where they regulate the balance between excitation and inhibition. CB2 receptors influence immune signaling and neuroinflammation.

Studies using brain imaging suggest that cannabinoids modulate glutamate and GABA signaling, processes often disrupted in autism spectrum presentations. This helps explain why some patients become calmer, sleep more consistently, and communicate more easily when supported with cannabinoid therapy.

GLOBAL CLINICAL EVIDENCE

Research from Israel, Brazil, Canada, Europe, and Australia has created a steadily growing body of evidence. In Israel, Dr. Adi Aran and colleagues evaluated CBD-rich preparations in children with severe behavioral challenges and found caregiver reported improvements in behavior, anxiety, and communication. A later interventional trial tested oral oil preparations with high CBD to THC ratios and confirmed tolerability along with promising signs of efficacy.

In Brazil, a prospective study of children receiving CBD-rich extracts reported improvements in social interaction, communication, behavior, and sleep. Families also reported reducing the need for other medications over time. Canadian and European registries describe similar real world results, with parents noting calmer routines, better rest, and lower agitation.

Recent systematic reviews pooling data from Israel and Brazil concluded that CBD formulations can reduce disruptive behavior, improve social responsiveness, and support sleep, while calling for larger randomized trials. Reviews published in 2024 and 2025 reinforced these conclusions, highlighting consistent signals of benefit and favorable safety profiles.

While most studies have focused on CBD-rich preparations for safety reasons, clinicians increasingly recognize that carefully balanced amounts of THC and other cannabinoids such as CBG or CBN may enhance therapeutic outcomes through the entourage effect. Early anecdotal reports suggest that these broader-spectrum formulations may support mood regulation, focus, and daily adaptability in ways CBD alone cannot fully achieve.

WHAT US AND UK RESEARCHERS ARE EXPLORING

In the United States, clinical work has focused on anxiety, irritability, and sleep, along with brain level measures of excitation and inhibition. Several ongoing trials are evaluating CBD in children and adults with autism, using standardized rating scales for irritability and social function.

In the United Kingdom, neuroimaging studies demonstrated that a single dose of CBD can shift neurotransmitter balance in the cortex. This mechanistic evidence aligns with caregiver reports of calmer behavior and improved stress tolerance.

SYMPTOMS THAT OFTEN IMPROVE

Families and researchers consistently report improvements across several domains. Irritability and aggression are reduced, with fewer outbursts and less self injury. Sleep becomes deeper and more predictable, which helps daytime behavior and learning. Social responsiveness improves, with more eye contact, smoother transitions, and greater engagement. Anxiety and sensory distress also decline, allowing children and adults to cope better with noise, crowds, and changes in routine.

FORMULATIONS AND PRACTICAL APPROACHES

Most programs begin with CBD-forward oils or capsules to provide steady daytime regulation. Small amounts of THC may be added for evening calm or persistent agitation. Oromucosal sprays and liquids allow precise titration, while terpene enriched oils are being tested for calming and sleep supportive effects. Vaporization is commonly used for rapid onset in certain cases, though less often in pediatric care. The common principle is careful adjustment to achieve more predictable days and peaceful nights.

COMORBID EPILEPSY AND OVERLAPPING BENEFITS

Many children and adults on the spectrum also live with seizure disorders. Evidence from epilepsy trials shows that CBD can reduce seizure frequency in specific syndromes, and families often report that fewer seizures and better sleep lead to improvements in behavior and learning. While autism is distinct from epilepsy, this overlap helps explain why cannabinoid care sometimes produces benefits across multiple areas of life.

WHAT THE LATEST REVIEWS SAY

Recent systematic reviews published in 2023, 2024, and 2025 converge on a consistent picture. CBD-rich formulations appear to reduce irritability and disruptive behavior, improve social responsiveness, and support sleep. Safety signals remain favorable in short to medium term studies. Authors emphasize the need for larger multi-center trials with standardized products and longer follow-up, but the direction of evidence is clear.

THE US CHALLENGE AND THE GLOBAL OPPORTUNITY

Families in the United States often discover Cannabis through state programs rather than coordinated medical systems. Federal restrictions have slowed large randomized trials and limited clinician training. By contrast, Israel has national programs that prospectively track outcomes, and Canada and parts of Europe have integrated standardized products into autism care. Australia is also expanding structured prescribing and monitoring.

This gap means American families are left to navigate largely on their own while high quality data accumulates abroad. Registered US trials are expanding, and several are now enrolling children and adults with focus on severe irritability, anxiety, and sleep disturbance.

PATIENT OUTCOMES AND FAMILY STORIES

Across studies and registries, the message is consistent. Cannabis does not simply change one symptom; it reshapes daily life. Parents describe calmer mornings, fewer crises during transitions, and nights where the whole household sleeps. Teachers notice more time on task and fewer disruptions. Adults on the spectrum report feeling more at ease in social settings and more able to communicate needs. Families speak of rediscovering rhythm and connection.

WHY THIS MATTERS

Autism is not one story but many. Each individual has unique strengths and struggles, and families often face exhausting journeys through fragmented care. Cannabis offers a path toward greater stability by calming the nervous system, supporting sleep, and improving the predictability of each day.

The global evidence from Israel, Brazil, Canada, Europe, and Australia points in the same direction: *CBD-rich formulations can* *reduce disruptive behaviors and improve social function, particularly when added to existing supports.*

The next steps are clear. Expand access to high quality products, support clinicians and families with education, and run large trials that match the scale of the need.

For children and adults on the spectrum, these changes mean more peaceful days, safer nights, and more opportunities to grow. Cannabis is not just symptom relief. It is a bridge toward dignity, stability, and potential.

19

SKIN & INFLAMMATION DISORDERS (DERMATITIS, ECZEMA & PSORIASIS)

UNDERSTANDING SKIN AND INFLAMMATION DISORDERS

The skin is the body's largest organ, and it often reflects the state of internal health. Conditions such as dermatitis, eczema, and psoriasis affect millions worldwide. In the United States, more than thirty-million people live with eczema and over seven-million with psoriasis. Globally, the World Health Organization estimates that psoriasis alone impacts two to three percent of the population.

These conditions bring redness, itching, flaking, and pain. They interfere with sleep, limit social participation, and often cause embarrassment. Because the symptoms are visible, the psychological burden is heavy. People living with eczema and psoriasis experience higher rates of anxiety, depression, and social withdrawal. Families carry the additional strain of ongoing dermatology appointments and the financial weight of expensive biologic therapies that can cost thousands of dollars each year.

THE ENDOCANNABINOID SYSTEM AND SKIN HEALTH

The skin contains an extensive network of endocannabinoid receptors. CB1 and CB2 are found in keratinocytes, sebaceous glands, hair follicles, and immune cells within the skin. Endocannabinoids such as anandamide regulate cell turnover, barrier function, and inflammatory responses.

When this system falls out of balance, skin conditions flare. Cannabinoids from the plant interact with these same pathways. CBD calms inflammatory signals and reduces itch. THC modifies pain perception. Other cannabinoids such as CBG and CBN demonstrate antibacterial and anti-inflammatory activity. Cannabinoids also influence TRPV1 receptors, which mediate sensations of itching and burning. This helps explain why many patients describe near-instant relief when applying CBD creams. Emerging evidence also shows that CBD supports skin-barrier repair by reducing water loss, which is a crucial factor in eczema.

RESEARCH EVIDENCE AROUND THE WORLD

Research from several regions confirms consistent benefits.

In the United States, small clinical studies show that CBD creams reduce itching and improve hydration in eczema patients. People with psoriasis who used topical cannabinoids reported less scaling, redness, and pain.

In Europe, Italian and German teams found that cannabinoid creams strengthened skin-barrier function and lowered inflammatory markers. Israeli medical Cannabis registries report widespread use of cannabinoid topicals for psoriasis, often combined with oral oils to address systemic inflammation.

Canada's observational studies echo these findings, with patients reporting itch relief, improved sleep, and less reliance on steroid creams. Preclinical studies add a mechanistic foundation, showing that cannabinoids normalize skin cell growth rates, reduce inflammatory cytokines, and calm immune overactivity.

Full-spectrum formulations that combine CBD with small amounts of THC appear to amplify these benefits. CBD calms inflammatory signaling and helps restore barrier integrity, while THC engages peripheral CB1 receptors to further ease local pain and itch. Used topically, these combinations do not produce intoxication, but patients consistently describe relief as deeper and longer-lasting than with CBD-only creams. Minor cannabinoids like CBG and select terpenes may add complementary effects.

A 2022 systematic review pooling data from the United States, Europe, and Israel concluded that cannabinoid topicals consistently reduced itch severity and skin dryness, while calling for larger randomized trials to strengthen the evidence base.

HOW CANNABIS HELPS IN DAILY LIFE

For patients, the benefits go far beyond the clinic. Cannabis creams relieve itch, calm redness, and soften plaques. CBD slows accelerated skin cell turnover in psoriasis, reducing scaling and discomfort. THC and CBD together relieve nerve-related burning sensations. With irritation calmed, sleep improves, and patients experience deeper rest. The psychological toll also lessens. Visible improvements in skin health reduce anxiety, ease social fears, and allow patients to re-engage with everyday life.

Parents of children with eczema often describe finally sleeping through the night because scratching and bleeding were reduced. Adults with psoriasis report feeling comfortable enough to wear short sleeves or shorts for the first time in years. One patient described being able to attend her daughter's wedding in a sleeveless dress without fear of judgment. Another spoke of returning to the beach with confidence after a decade of hiding his skin. These are victories of dignity as much as of health.

FORMULATIONS AND APPROACHES

Patients and clinics use a range of Cannabis formulations. Topical creams and balms are applied directly to plaques, rashes, or inflamed areas. Oils and tinctures provide systemic support for widespread inflammation. THC-infused topicals reduce pain and itching without causing intoxication, as they rarely enter the bloodstream in significant amounts. Combination products that blend CBD, THC, and minor cannabinoids provide broader relief. Terpenes such as linalool and beta-caryophyllene enhance anti-inflammatory action, while limonene adds antimicrobial support. Emerging transdermal patches and gels offer longer lasting delivery for chronic conditions.

Consistency is key. Patients often find the greatest relief when creams are applied regularly after bathing or moisturizing.

THE UNITED STATES CHALLENGE VS GLOBAL PROGRESS

In the United States, Cannabis topicals are widely available in state programs but lack FDA approval. This limits physician guidance and leaves patients to experiment on their own. Insurance coverage is rare, making long term treatment costly for families. Federal restrictions have also slowed the pace of large clinical trials.

In contrast, Israel, Europe, and Canada are actively integrating cannabinoids into dermatology. Structured studies, licensed topical products, and national registries have produced higher quality data abroad than in the United States. Australia is also expanding prescriptions for skin disorders as demand grows.

POLICY AND ACCESS

Skin disorders are not life threatening, but their impact is profound. Policymakers often overlook them when deciding qualifying conditions. Yet millions of people live with chronic itch, pain, and stigma. Expanding research and improving access to cannabinoid therapies would provide safe and effective relief for a vast population.

Equity in care matters. Patients with skin disorders are too often dismissed because their conditions are not fatal, even though the toll on mental health, work, and family is immense.

WHY THIS MATTERS

Dermatitis, eczema, and psoriasis are not cosmetic concerns but chronic inflammatory disorders that affect health, comfort, and dignity. Cannabis has proven to be one of the few therapies that can calm the itch, reduce redness, restore rest, and bring relief without the side effects of steroids or biologics.

This matters because skin disorders are visible in every sense. They are visible on the body, visible in the distress they cause, and visible in the way society overlooks them. Cannabis changes this story. It restores confidence, reduces suffering, and allows people to feel whole in their own skin again.

Cannabis is not only a balm for the skin. It is a balm for the spirit, helping people reclaim comfort, confidence, and quality of life.

Cannabis is not only a balm for the skin; it is a balm for the spirit, restoring comfort, confidence, and quality of life.

20

OTHER EMERGING CONDITIONS (ALS, TOURETTE'S, BONE HEALTH & MORE)

WHY EMERGING CONDITIONS MATTER

Cannabis has already proven its value in conditions such as pain, epilepsy, cancer, and multiple sclerosis. Yet science continues to uncover benefits in diseases that once seemed far beyond the reach of plant based medicine. These emerging conditions are where innovation, research, and patient courage come together. Families often turn to Cannabis as a last resort, and the results they report have inspired entire new lines of research around the world.

Emerging conditions are also where patients lead science. Veterans, parents, and grassroots advocates often move forward where policy and medicine stall. This frontier represents not only the next wave of Cannabis medicine, but also the breaking down of stigma as real lives are changed.

AMYOTROPHIC LATERAL SCLEROSIS (ALS)

ALS, also known as Lou Gehrig's disease, is one of the most devastating neurological conditions. It is marked by the steady loss of motor neurons, leaving patients unable to walk, speak, and eventually breathe. There is no cure. Current treatments slow progression slightly, but symptoms such as spasticity, pain, and appetite loss often remain uncontrolled.

Cannabis has offered relief where standard options fall short. Studies in the United States and Europe show that Cannabis can reduce spasticity, improve sleep, and restore appetite. Preclinical work suggests that cannabinoids may protect neurons from excitotoxicity and oxidative stress, two processes strongly linked to motor neuron death.

Patients often describe not only physical relief but also a sense of calm, which is critical in a disease that can leave people feeling trapped in their own bodies. Some say Cannabis made swallowing easier, reduced choking episodes, or allowed them to sleep through the night for the first time in months. Families describe less tension and more peaceful moments together. The ALS Association has acknowledged these reports, even as formal clinical guidance remains cautious.

TOURETTE'S SYNDROME

Tourette's syndrome is defined by involuntary motor and vocal tics that can be disruptive and socially stigmatizing. Standard medicines include antipsychotics and sedatives, but these often bring side effects such as weight gain, drowsiness, and mood changes.

Cannabis has offered a new path forward. German and Israeli studies, including double blind controlled trials, have shown that THC can significantly reduce the frequency and intensity of tics. In some cases, patients reported near complete suppression of tics within minutes of dosing.

CBD has been studied as well, with mixed but encouraging results for anxiety, sleep, and stress management. Many Tourette's patients also live with comorbid conditions such as obsessive compulsive disorder, ADHD, and generalized anxiety. Cannabis often helps with these overlapping struggles, bringing a more comprehensive form of relief.

Patients describe Cannabis as restoring dignity and confidence in social situations. Some report being able to return to work or school without constant fear of embarrassment. Families notice calmer evenings, smoother routines, and more consistent sleep. For many, Cannabis has meant not just fewer tics but the chance to live without stigma.

BONE HEALTH AND OSTEOPOROSIS

Bones are not static structures. They are living tissue that constantly break down and rebuild in a cycle of renewal. Osteoporosis and other bone disorders occur when breakdown exceeds repair. The result is fragile bones, fractures, and a serious loss of independence.

Osteoporosis affects one in three women and one in five men over the age of fifty worldwide.

The Endocannabinoid System is deeply involved in bone biology. CB2 receptors are abundant in bone, where they regulate the balance between osteoblasts, which build bone, and osteoclasts, which break it down. Animal studies have shown that cannabinoids stimulate bone formation, slow bone loss, and improve fracture healing. In humans, observational studies suggest Cannabis users may have stronger bone density, though results vary depending on lifestyle and other factors. More compelling is evidence that cannabinoids may speed fracture healing by stimulating bone formation directly. This has been documented in animal studies and hinted at in case reports of patients who healed faster than expected.

For elderly patients or those at risk of osteoporosis, Cannabis represents a new frontier in care. It may help prevent fractures, reduce pain from brittle bones, and improve quality of life. Considering the massive global burden of osteoporosis, even small benefits would translate to millions of people living longer, healthier, and more independent lives.

NEURODEGENERATIVE DISORDERS BEYOND ALZHEIMER'S AND PARKINSON'S

Cannabis has also shown promise in several other progressive brain disorders. In Huntington's disease, small trials suggest cannabinoids reduce involuntary movements known as chorea, while also improving behavior and sleep. Families describe calmer daily routines and less emotional strain.

In frontotemporal dementia, caregivers in Europe report that Cannabis oils reduce agitation and aggression, easing household tension. In the rare and devastating Creutzfeldt Jakob disease, Cannabis has been used to bring comfort by reducing pain, easing spasms, and supporting sleep in the final stages of illness.

While research is limited, these conditions highlight how cannabinoids act broadly across the nervous system. Patients and families often emphasize that Cannabis provides not only symptom relief but also meaningful improvements in quality of life during some of the most difficult diagnoses.

AUTOIMMUNE AND INFLAMMATORY DISORDERS

Beyond arthritis and Crohn's disease, Cannabis is being explored for other immune related conditions. In lupus, patients report fewer flares, less fatigue, and reductions in pain. Preclinical studies suggest cannabinoids reduce autoantibody production, calming the immune system without shutting it down entirely.

In scleroderma, early evidence indicates that Cannabis may reduce skin tightening and improve circulation. In myasthenia gravis, limited reports suggest improvements in muscle fatigue and endurance.

The strength of Cannabis in autoimmune disease lies in its ability to modulate the immune system without fully suppressing it. Unlike standard immunosuppressants, which increase infection risk, cannabinoids appear to rebalance immune activity in a gentler way. Patient advocacy groups are already lobbying for expanded access and more research in these overlooked conditions.

NEUROPATHIC DISORDERS AND PAIN SYNDROMES

Cannabis has already shown clear benefit in fibromyalgia, migraines, and diabetic neuropathy, but other pain syndromes also deserve attention. In phantom limb pain, veterans and amputees report relief when no other therapy helped.

In complex regional pain syndrome, one of the most difficult chronic pain conditions to treat, Cannabis helps calm nerve driven pain and restore sleep. In chemotherapy induced neuropathy, cannabinoids reduce both nerve pain and nausea, offering a twofold benefit for patients undergoing cancer treatment.

These conditions underscore one of the greatest strengths of Cannabis. It often succeeds where opioids fail, providing relief without the same risks of dependency or overdose.

SKIN DISORDERS BEYOND ECZEMA AND PSORIASIS

Cannabis is also being studied in other dermatologic conditions. In acne, CBD reduces oil production in sebaceous glands and calms inflammation. Early clinical studies show fewer breakouts and less redness.

In vitiligo, where patches of skin lose pigment, small studies suggest cannabinoids may support repigmentation when combined with light therapy. Improvements in visible skin appearance often translate into restored confidence and reduced social stigma.

In wound healing, cannabinoid creams have shown faster closure and less scarring in preclinical research. Patients using these preparations report less pain during dressing changes and better cosmetic outcomes.

CANCER BEYOND SYMPTOM RELIEF

While earlier chapters addressed Cannabis for symptom management in cancer, emerging evidence points to possible direct anti-tumor effects. Laboratory studies show that cannabinoids can slow the growth of glioblastoma, breast cancer, and pancreatic cancer cells.

Clinical trials in Europe are now testing THC and CBD as adjuncts to chemotherapy. While these studies are still in early stages, they represent one of the most exciting directions in oncology research. It is important to emphasize that Cannabis should not be seen as a replacement for standard therapies, but as a complement that may enhance treatment effectiveness while also supporting quality of life.

RARE AND PEDIATRIC CONDITIONS

Some of the most moving stories in Cannabis medicine come from rare and pediatric conditions. In Dravet syndrome and Lennox-Gastaut syndrome, CBD is already FDA approved as Epidiolex to reduce seizures. Families describe this therapy as life changing, transforming children's daily function and providing hope where once there was none.

In fragile X syndrome, cannabinoid trials show improvements in anxiety, irritability, and social interaction. In Rett syndrome, preclinical studies suggest neuroprotective benefits, and early human trials are underway.

These cases remind us why compassionate access matters. For families facing rare diseases with no effective options, Cannabis provides not only symptom relief but also a chance at stability, dignity, and hope.

THE UNITED STATES CHALLENGE VS GLOBAL PROGRESS

Once again, the United States lags behind global leaders in Cannabis research. Israeli scientists conduct some of the most advanced clinical trials in autism, epilepsy, and neurodegeneration. European and Canadian researchers steadily publish data on conditions such as Tourette's and bone health. Meanwhile, many American patients are left to experiment through state programs without the benefit of structured clinical oversight.

This is not because of lack of science but because of policy. Federal restrictions have slowed the pace of discovery, leaving American families behind even as other nations move ahead.

WHY THIS MATTERS

Cannabis helps across emerging conditions in profound ways. It reduces inflammation, protects neurons from oxidative stress, restores sleep and appetite, reduces pain and spasticity, and brings calm to anxious minds. While it is not a cure, across dozens of conditions it consistently improves quality of life in ways few medicines can match.

This matters because patients with ALS, Tourette's, osteoporosis, lupus, rare syndromes, and countless other diagnoses are too often told that nothing more can be done. Cannabis offers them something to try, something to hope for, and in many cases, something that works.

For the United States, embracing this frontier means investing in trials, building compassionate access, and catching up to nations already proving what is possible. For patients and families, it means fewer nights of despair, more days of comfort, and renewed faith in the power of science and nature together.

Cannabis is not only for the conditions we know well. It is for the conditions we are still discovering. It is not only a medicine of the present. It is a medicine of the future.

Cannabis offers them something to try, something to hope for, and in many cases, something that works.

CANNABIS ACROSS LIFE STAGES & SOCIETY

"Cannabis does not belong to one age, one diagnosis, or one demographic; it follows the human life cycle, meeting people where they are, when they need it most."

21

CANNABIS AND CHILDREN

THE SILENT VOICES

Children are the most vulnerable among us. They rely on adults, medicine, and society to protect them. Yet when it comes to medical Cannabis, children in the United States have been some of the most neglected patients. They are shielded from many dangers in life, yet when a plant with the power to help is within reach, the law itself becomes the barrier.

Around the world, research shows Cannabis can relieve seizures, ease cancer symptoms, reduce chronic pain, calm autism spectrum challenges, and bring comfort to children with rare genetic disorders. But in the United States, families often face barriers that force them to uproot their lives, cross state lines, or risk arrest simply to help their child.

A child born with leukemia or epilepsy does not know the life they are missing. Hospitals and medications become their normal. Adults diagnosed later in life remember what health felt like, but children born into illness never get that chance. They deserve every tool available to ease their suffering and give them dignity, comfort, and the possibility of better days.

THE ENDOCANNABINOID SYSTEM IN CHILDREN

Children, like adults, have an Endocannabinoid System. This natural network regulates sleep, appetite, mood, and immunity. When it is imbalanced, conditions such as epilepsy, autism, and cancer-related pain become harder to control. Plant-derived cannabinoids can help restore balance.

CBD has been studied most extensively in children. The FDA approval of Epidiolex, a CBD-based medicine for Dravet and Lennox-Gastaut syndromes, was a landmark moment.

It proved what parents had been saying for decades: *Cannabis can spare children from endless seizures when nothing else works.*

That approval was more than regulatory; it was a moral acknowledgment. It validated the voices of families who fought stigma, endured judgment, and demanded compassion. It showed that science must follow where patients lead.

CONDITIONS WHERE CANNABIS HELPS CHILDREN

Epilepsy: *Childhood epilepsy, especially syndromes like Dravet and Lennox-Gastaut, can bring hundreds of seizures each week.*

Each seizure robs development and quality of life. Medicines often fail or cause unbearable side effects. Epidiolex reduced seizures by more than 40 percent, with some children nearly seizure free. Beyond the United States, studies in Israel and Brazil have published studies showing CBD oils not only reduce seizures but also improve alertness, sleep, and mood. Parents describe seeing their child's personality return. Epilepsy remains the clearest case that Cannabis is both safe and transformative for children.

Cancer: *For children with cancer, chemotherapy is often as punishing as the disease itself.*

Nausea, vomiting, weight loss, and pain strip away strength and joy. Cannabis restores appetite, eases pain, and calms nausea. In Israel and Canada, pediatric oncology wards integrate Cannabis oils into care. Families describe children smiling, playing, and eating again. In the United States, many parents often turn to dispensaries without physician guidance, left to navigate alone. This divide is not about science but about politics.

Autism Spectrum Disorder: *Autism brings challenges in behavior, communication, and sleep.*

Families often endure daily aggression, self injury, and exhaustion. Clinical trials in Israel have shown CBD-rich oils significantly reduce anxiety, calm behavior, and improve sleep. Similar findings in Brazil and Canada echo these results. Parents say Cannabis gives them their child back. Teachers see calmer classrooms. Siblings finally get to play without fear. These outcomes are not small, they change the fabric of daily family life.

Rare Genetic Disorders: *Fragile X, Rett syndrome, and other rare conditions combine seizures, developmental delays, and anxiety.*

CBD trials in Fragile X show reduced irritability and social avoidance. In Rett syndrome, early research points to neuroprotection and seizure reduction. For families with few options, Cannabis becomes a lifeline that restores stability to otherwise chaotic lives.

Pain and Palliative Care: *For children with terminal illnesses or chronic pain, Cannabis offers dignity and comfort.*

It eases suffering in muscular dystrophy, rare metabolic disorders, and pediatric cancers. In Canada and Israel, palliative teams use Cannabis to reduce opioids and restore quality of life. Families speak of finally having meaningful time together instead of watching their child suffer in silence.

PATIENT STORIES THAT CHANGED THE DEBATE

Charlotte Figi, a young girl with Dravet syndrome, became a global symbol when CBD oil dramatically reduced her seizures. Her story sparked a movement, opening hearts and shifting laws.

Her story broke into national consciousness in 2013 through Dr. Sanjay Gupta's *WEED* documentary, capturing headlines and sparking conversation. Her case opened hearts and shifted laws. But Charlotte was only one of thousands. In the years since, thousands of families have reported similar turnarounds, building a body of lived evidence that helped reshape state policies and clinical practice.

Across the United States, parents have risked everything; careers, homes, even custody, to fight for access. They became advocates not because they wanted to, but because their children left them no choice.

WHY POLICY MUST CHANGE

The science is no longer in question. The stories are no longer rare. The need is no longer debatable.

A handful of states, including Colorado and California, have taken steps toward pediatric integration and yet, national leadership across the United States as a whole, continues to fail its children by remaining absent.

Other nations have acted with compassion and urgency. Israel built national pediatric Cannabis programs where families receive guidance, dosing protocols, and physician oversight. Canada regulates safe, standardized oils and integrates them into pediatric oncology and neurology wards. Across Europe, governments fund clinical trials and collect real world data so families are not left to guess.

Meanwhile, American families are abandoned to a patchwork of inconsistent state laws. Some parents can access Cannabis for their child in one state but face criminal charges if they cross a border to another state. Insurance refuses to cover medicine, leaving desperate families to drain savings. Physicians fear professional backlash, so many stay silent even when they believe Cannabis could help.

This is not a policy gap. It is systemic neglect. Every untreated seizure, every night of agony, every child who dies without comfort is not only a tragedy but also a failure of leadership. Lawmakers, like the current Lt. Governor Dan Patrick of Texas, speak endlessly about protecting children, yet allow politics and stigma to override actual compassion and science. He is not the only one. Across the country, from state to state, voices like his echo all the way to Washington, where ancient beliefs continue to hold our children hostage.

How many more Charlottes must there be before leaders act? How many families must become refugees within their own country, moving across state lines to save their child? How many children must die knowing relief existed but was denied because adults in power looked away?

History will not forgive this. One day, when Cannabis is integrated into pediatric care as seamlessly as antibiotics or insulin, society will look back and ask why we forced children to suffer while the evidence was already in our hands. Those who chose inaction will have no defense.

WHY THIS MATTERS

This chapter is not about abstract debates or political talking points. It is about children whose lives are measured in seizures, hospital stays, and moments of pain that never should have been allowed.

It matters because a child with epilepsy who seizes hundreds of times a week deserves more than sympathy; they deserve every tool modern medicine can offer. It matters because a child with cancer should not vomit day after day when a plant could bring them comfort and strength. It matters because children with autism, Fragile X, or Rett syndrome deserve calm, connection, and dignity, not endless cycles of failed pharmaceuticals.

It matters because these are children who do not get a second childhood. Every year lost to seizures, pain, or sleepless nights is a year they will never get back. Families cannot wait decades for bureaucracy to catch up.

This matters not only for the children but for the parents who sit awake every night listening for a seizure monitor, for the siblings who live in constant fear, for the grandparents who watch helplessly as another generation suffers. When Cannabis restores rest, when it brings back a smile, when it allows a family to share a meal together in peace, it is not simply medicine, it is restoration of humanity itself.

It matters because a society is judged not by how it treats its wealthiest or its strongest, but by how it cares for its most vulnerable. And right now, America is failing that test.

Cannabis will not cure every disease. But it can give children dignity, comfort, and hope. It can give parents the gift of seeing their child's laughter return. It can give families the peace of knowing they did everything possible. That is why this matters. That is why delay is unacceptable. That is why change cannot wait.

When a child is suffering and relief exists, denying access is not caution; it is neglect.

22

TALKING TO TEENS ABOUT CANNABIS

THE FIRST CONVERSATIONS

For many, the first time Cannabis is mentioned is not in a doctor's office or in a medical journal. Middle school is often when teens first hear about Cannabis, sometimes from peers who are curious, sometimes from older siblings, and sometimes from the internet.

This makes it essential for parents to begin conversations early. Teens deserve honesty, not scare tactics. Parents who explain the realities of Cannabis, its medical uses, and its risks give their children the tools to think critically instead of relying on myths shared by social media.

PEER PRESSURE AND INFLUENCE

Teenagers live in a world shaped heavily by their peers. Curiosity is natural, and pressure to experiment can feel overwhelming. Parents cannot control every environment their children walk into, but they can prepare them for those moments. Preparation begins long before exposure, in honest, age-appropriate talks that normalize questions instead of punishing them. When teens understand Cannabis as a plant with medical potential but also as something that can be misused if started too early, they are better equipped to make thoughtful decisions.

Conversations should also acknowledge that Cannabis is not the only substance teens will encounter. Alcohol, vaping, and other drugs are present in their world. Placing Cannabis in context helps them see it for what it is, not what others exaggerate it to be.

One of the biggest risks parents face is allowing misinformation to take hold. If Cannabis is portrayed as more dangerous than it actually is, teens may later dismiss parental advice entirely. But if parents are open and truthful, teens are more likely to trust them and pause before making risky choices.

THE ROLE OF PARENTS

The responsibility of guiding teens rests with parents and guardians. Teens listen more than they admit, and they notice when parents remain silent. By setting a tone of open discussion, parents can reduce stigma and create trust. When a teen feels safe asking questions, the conversation becomes a learning opportunity rather than a lecture.

Parents should emphasize that legal age matters, just as it does for alcohol and tobacco. Cannabis can help patients with medical conditions, but recreational use is restricted for a reason. Framing it as an issue of health, maturity, and responsibility rather than morality or punishment, helps teens understand the difference.

Parents do not need all the answers to be effective. Simply listening, validating concerns, and encouraging dialogue often matters more than delivering a perfect speech.

THE CONFUSING PATCHWORK OF LAWS

One of the hardest parts for teenagers to grasp is the inconsistency of Cannabis laws. In some states, Cannabis is legal and celebrated. In others, possession of even a small amount can result in arrest, criminal charges, and a permanent record.

Even adults struggle to navigate this patchwork of laws, so it's no surprise that teens find it confusing. Teens need to hear from parents that while Cannabis may be accepted in some places, it remains illegal for them as minors everywhere. The goal is not to instill fear, but to emphasize safety, legality, and the importance of waiting until the right time.

In Colorado, a 21 year old can walk into a dispensary and buy Cannabis legally. In Texas, the same plant leads to jail time. Teens deserve to understand these contrasts clearly.

TALKING POINTS FOR PARENTS

Parents can stress that Cannabis is a plant with medical value but not something safe for recreational use during adolescence. Just because a friend has a prescription does not make it legal or safe to share. Laws vary widely, and what is permitted in one state may bring serious consequences in another.

Above all, growing up means learning to make choices. Parents are not judges, but guides in that process.

WHY THIS MATTERS

Teenagers today grow up in a world where Cannabis is far more visible than in the past. They see dispensaries on city streets, hear politicians debate legalization, and scroll past memes online celebrating 420. Without guidance, it is easy for them to be misled.

Talking to teens about Cannabis is not about scaring them. It is about preparing them. It is about giving them facts instead of myths, and respect instead of judgment. Teens who hear the truth from their parents are more likely to pause, reflect, and make decisions that keep them safe.

As we move from the world of teens to that of adults, another group faces unique struggles with Cannabis: *our veterans.*

23

VETERANS AND CANNABIS

THE COST OF SERVICE

More than eighteen million veterans live in the United States today. Nearly five million carry lasting disabilities from their service. Behind every number is a person who gave part of their body, their mind, or their spirit in service to the nation. Some lost limbs in battle. Others returned with chronic pain that never leaves. Many carry invisible wounds like post traumatic stress that linger long after combat ends.

America honors veterans with parades, flags, and speeches. But when the ceremonies end, many are left to navigate a system that is underfunded, slow, and often indifferent. The same country that trusted them with weapons of war too often fails to provide real healing when they come home. Veterans have proven themselves time and again. Yet the medicine that many say has saved their lives is still out of reach within the very system that was built to serve them.

THE WEIGHT OF TRAUMA

Post-traumatic stress disorder affects nearly one in five veterans from recent conflicts, and for Vietnam veterans the number has reached as high as thirty percent. PTSD is not a passing struggle. It is a constant state of fear and hypervigilance. Veterans describe waking in cold sweats from nightmares, scanning restaurants for exits, or reliving battlefield moments at the sound of a car backfiring.

The VA has relied heavily on antidepressants, anti-anxiety medications, and opioids. These drugs often numb emotions without addressing the root of the trauma. Many veterans turn to alcohol to dull the pain, which leads to broken families and addiction.

Cannabis offers a different path. Studies in New Mexico and Colorado documented veterans using Cannabis with fewer intrusive memories, longer sleep, and reduced anxiety. The American Legion conducted a national survey where more than ninety percent of veterans supported research into Cannabis for PTSD and pain. Veterans groups have said again and again that Cannabis gives them relief where nothing else has.

CHRONIC PAIN AND LOST LIMBS

Since 2001, more than sixteen hundred United States service members have returned with major limb amputations. Tens of thousands more live with back injuries, joint damage, and nerve pain from deployments, combat loads, and blast impacts. Chronic pain is one of the most common reasons veterans seek care at the VA, which remains one of the largest prescribers of opioids in the nation.

These pills are handed out quickly, but the results are tragic. Veterans are twice as likely as civilians to die from opioid overdose. Cannabis has proven to be a safer alternative. Studies show that veterans who use Cannabis reduce their opioid intake by more than half, with many able to stop completely.

Phantom limb pain is one of the hardest conditions to treat with conventional medicine. Veterans describe Cannabis calming the burning, stabbing sensations that opioids never touched. One veteran said, *"For the first time since I lost my leg, I can sleep without waking from the pain."* Others describe using Cannabis topicals or edibles to regain the ability to walk, rest, and live without constant agony.

TRAUMATIC BRAIN INJURY AND HEALING

Modern warfare has left a legacy of brain injuries. More than 450,000 service members have been diagnosed with traumatic brain injury since 2000. Symptoms include memory loss, mood swings, difficulty focusing, and chronic headaches. Many veterans describe feeling like different people after their injuries, struggling to maintain relationships or employment.

Cannabinoids have shown potential as neuroprotective agents. Research suggests they can reduce brain inflammation, limit cell damage, and improve recovery of function. TBI is often called the signature wound of modern war, and Cannabis offers a line of hope where traditional therapies fail. Veterans themselves testify that Cannabis helps them stabilize mood, control headaches, and find calm when nothing else has worked.

THE SUICIDE CRISIS

Every day, an average of twenty veterans die by suicide. That is more than six thousand lives lost each year. Since 9/11, more veterans have died from suicide than in combat. This is not just a national crisis but a complete moral failure.

The VA's own reports confirm that veterans face a suicide rate fifty percent higher than civilians. Risk is highest among younger veterans who served in Iraq and Afghanistan. Families are left grieving loved ones who survived war but could not survive coming home.

Cannabis is not a cure, but many veterans credit it with keeping them alive. It allows them to sleep, to escape nightmares, to ease pain, and to reconnect with family. One Marine veteran told Congress, "I would not be here today if it were not for Cannabis." Denying this option is not just poor policy, it is cruelty. Families who have buried veterans know this pain too well, and many have become advocates pushing for Cannabis reform so that others will not face the same loss.

THE FAILURE OF THE VA AND FEDERAL POLICY

The Department of Veterans Affairs is bound by federal law. That means VA doctors cannot prescribe Cannabis and cannot even recommend it, even in states where it is fully legal. Veterans who want access must leave the VA system and pay out of pocket. Meanwhile, opioids are covered and handed out freely.

Several bipartisan bills have been introduced to allow VA doctors to discuss Cannabis with patients. Again and again, these bills have stalled. Politicians praise veterans in public but fail to act when it comes to real change. Veterans are left to navigate a maze of state laws, often spending hundreds each month for medicine they should have access to through their earned benefits.

THE HYPOCRISY OF AMERICAN LEADERSHIP

The hypocrisy is impossible to ignore. In Washington, politicians sit in air-conditioned offices surrounded by security details, far removed from the chaos of war. Their biggest risks are losing votes or committee seats. Yet when veterans return home asking for help, many of those same politicians block access to Cannabis.

They stand behind podiums on Veterans Day declaring *"support our troops,"* but in the halls of Congress they allow bills to stall, hearings to vanish into bureaucracy, and policies to remain frozen in stigma. They wave flags in parades while denying the medicine that veterans say has saved their lives.

Other nations have already moved forward. Canada provides Cannabis to veterans through its national health system. Israel integrates Cannabis directly into military and veteran care, where doctors prescribe it openly for PTSD and chronic pain. Europe funds clinical trials and collects long term outcomes. These countries act not because they have more resources, but because they have more compassion.

The United States, with all its wealth and medical power, continues to fail. Veterans who fought for freedom abroad are denied freedom at home. They must leave the VA system, spend hundreds out of pocket, and navigate dispensaries without medical guidance, all while opioids and sedatives remain covered and readily prescribed.

This is not only policy failure. It is moral cowardice. Every day of political delay means another veteran suicide, another family grieving, another soldier betrayed. History will not remember the speeches or the parades. It will remember that when veterans asked for healing, too many leaders chose politics over people.

VOICES OF VETERANS

Veterans themselves are leading the fight for change. The Veterans Cannabis Project, Wounded Warrior initiatives, and state level organizations amplify their stories. Their voices are clear and consistent.

One Iraq veteran explained that Cannabis allowed him to put down the bottle and reconnect with his children. A Vietnam veteran said Cannabis was the only thing that quieted fifty years of nightmares. A Marine amputee shared that Cannabis topicals gave him back the ability to walk without burning pain. A female Army medic said Cannabis helped her manage both PTSD and migraines so she could return to school and build a new life.

These are not isolated stories. They are repeated across every state, from Vietnam veterans to Iraq and Afghanistan veterans. Cannabis is giving life back where the system has taken it away.

WHY THIS MATTERS

When a country asks people to risk their lives, it carries a sacred obligation to care for them when they come home. That obligation does not end at the battlefield. It extends to hospital rooms, therapy sessions, and family kitchens where healing should begin.

Cannabis is not just about medicine. For veterans, it is about dignity, survival, and justice.

This matters because veterans should never have to beg for relief. They should not be forced to choose between breaking the law or suffering in silence. They should not have to march into legislatures or testify before Congress simply to gain access to a plant that could save their lives. A nation that trusts them with weapons of war should trust them with Cannabis.

It matters because suicide should not be the leading cause of death for those who wore the uniform. The United States spends billions on defense budgets but refuses to fund research and access that could prevent veteran suicides. Every death is a policy failure. Every loss is proof that words like "*support our troops*" mean nothing without action.

It matters because honoring service means more than speeches and parades, it means action compassion, and accountability. It means listening to the men and women who served, respecting their voices, and providing them with the tools they know can help. Canada and

Israel have proven Cannabis can be integrated into veteran care safely and effectively. The United States has no excuse for delay.

Finally, it matters because veterans are not asking for luxury. They are asking for sleep without nightmares, days without crippling pain, and lives without constant trauma. They are asking to live. Cannabis can help provide that. The science is clear, the stories are powerful, and the need is urgent.

The question is not whether Cannabis should be an option for veterans. The question is why it is still being denied. History will not look kindly on the leaders who allowed politics to outweigh the lives of those who sacrificed for their country. And as we move forward, it is impossible not to notice that while Cannabis is denied, alcohol is celebrated in military and veteran culture. The next chapter will explore this contradiction directly.

A nation that trusts its soldiers with weapons of war should trust its veterans with Cannabis.

24

CANNABIS VS ALCOHOL

THE DOUBLE STANDARD

In the United States, alcohol is celebrated. It sponsors sporting events, fills grocery store aisles, and is woven into milestones from birthdays to weddings. Toasts mark promotions, holidays, and retirements. Alcohol is so deeply normalized that questioning its danger feels almost taboo.

Yet alcohol is one of the leading causes of preventable death, contributing to more than one hundred forty-thousand deaths per year in the United States alone. It fuels liver disease, heart conditions, neurological decline, and countless violent incidents.

Cannabis, by contrast, remains stigmatized and restricted, even though it is safer by every measurable standard. No one has ever died from a Cannabis overdose. It does not cause liver failure, does not damage the heart in the same way alcohol does, and does not drive violence or aggression. The double standard is glaring. One substance destroys lives yet is celebrated; the other heals lives yet remains criminalized.

HEALTH IMPACTS COMPARED

Alcohol damages nearly every organ system. It is directly tied to liver cirrhosis, multiple forms of cancer, cardiovascular disease, pancreatitis, and progressive neurological decline. Long-term use fuels depression and anxiety, creating a destructive cycle of dependency. It weakens the immune system, impairs judgment, and accelerates aging.

Cannabis shows the opposite profile, supporting the body through the Endocannabinoid System, reducing inflammation, regulating sleep, calming anxiety, and easing chronic pain. Where alcohol tears the body down, Cannabis restores balance.

Most striking of all, there has never been a single confirmed death anywhere in the world caused directly by Cannabis overdose. Alcohol poisoning kills thousands every year. Alcohol is toxic by its very nature. Cannabis continues to show promise in managing conditions ranging from epilepsy to arthritis to cancer-related symptoms.

SOCIAL CONSEQUENCES

Alcohol is one of the strongest drivers of violence in American society. It is a major factor in domestic abuse, violent crime, and sexual assault. Every year, tens of thousands of lives are lost on American roads because of alcohol impaired driving. Behind each statistic are shattered families, traumatized children, and scarred communities.

Cannabis does not fuel aggression. Most studies show it reduces hostility and promotes calm. In states where Cannabis has been legalized, alcohol related traffic fatalities have declined. Cannabis offers a safer social alternative, one that could reduce some of the worst harms alcohol has inflicted on society.

ADDICTION AND RECOVERY

Alcohol is one of the most addictive substances available. Withdrawal can be so severe that it is life threatening. Entire industries exist to treat alcohol dependency, and yet relapse rates remain high. Families are torn apart as loved ones cycle through detox and relapse again and again.

Cannabis offers something different. While it is not free of dependency risk, its profile is far safer. Many people use Cannabis to reduce alcohol intake, to move away from opioids, and to stabilize recovery. Substitution programs have documented thousands of cases where Cannabis helped people step back from destructive drinking patterns. Families witness firsthand how Cannabis supports balance, calm, and restoration where alcohol never could.

ECONOMIC COSTS

The economic burden of alcohol in the United States exceeds two hundred forty-billion dollars every year. These costs stem from healthcare, lost productivity, accidents, and the criminal justice system. Tax revenue from alcohol sales does not come close to offsetting the damage. Society absorbs the losses in hospital bills, welfare costs, foster placements, and funerals.

Cannabis, on the other hand, generates billions in tax revenue for states that regulate it. Legal Cannabis has reduced costs related to opioid overdoses, alcohol misuse, and law enforcement resources spent on prohibition. When managed responsibly, Cannabis is proving not only safer but also more economically beneficial. Where alcohol drains public systems, Cannabis contributes to them.

POLITICS AND HYPOCRISY

Why is alcohol fully legal while Cannabis remains restricted? The answer is not public safety. It is politics, money, and stigma.

For decades, alcohol companies have poured millions into lobbying against Cannabis legalization, fearful of losing market share. Politicians who benefit from campaign contributions often ignore scientific evidence and repeat outdated rhetoric. The result is a system that protects a dangerous industry while criminalizing a safer alternative.

The hypocrisy is glaring. If public health were truly the priority, Cannabis would have been legalized long ago and alcohol would face stricter controls. Instead, leaders protect an industry that profits from addiction and disease while blocking access to a plant that offers healing.

WHY THIS MATTERS

Cannabis and alcohol are not equal. One destroys; the other heals. One kills quietly; in hospitals, on highways, and in homes across America. The other offers relief, restoration, and balance to millions suffering from chronic conditions.

This matters because families continue to bury loved ones lost to alcohol. It matters because young adults are encouraged to drink at college parties yet punished for choosing Cannabis. It matters because science, compassion, and common sense demand change.

It matters for justice. Alcohol has been normalized through privilege, profit, and politics; Cannabis has been criminalized in ways that have devastated communities. The double standard has not only been deadly, it has been discriminatory.

It matters for economics. Billions are wasted treating alcohol related disease, while Cannabis revenues fund education, healthcare, and infrastructure in states that regulate it responsibly.

It matters for culture. Alcohol has been allowed to weave itself into every holiday, celebration, and ritual. Cannabis remains burdened by stigma, yet it is safer, gentler, and more beneficial.

History will not remember this era kindly. It will remember lawmakers who knew the truth but chose to maintain hypocrisy. It will remember the lives lost to alcohol while Cannabis remained locked behind stigma and law.

Cannabis offers a safer, smarter, and more compassionate path forward. The only question is whether leaders will have the courage to admit it and act.

Alcohol is celebrated despite the lives it destroys, while Cannabis is punished despite the lives it heals.

25

RECREATIONAL CANNABIS

A NEW ERA OF FREEDOM

For the first time in modern American history, adults can walk into brightly lit dispensaries, browse shelves of carefully cultivated Cannabis, and purchase it legally. What once was an act of defiance, carrying the risk of arrest and lifelong criminal records, has become an act of freedom. Recreational Cannabis represents more than a market. It represents choice, dignity, and the unraveling of decades of failed prohibition.

This new era is not only about access. It is about rewriting a narrative that cast millions of ordinary people as criminals for using a plant safer than alcohol. Legalization is the triumph of citizens over stigma, of evidence over fear, and of progress over punishment.

THE FEDERAL CONTRADICTION

Even as more than half of US states have legalized Cannabis for adult use, the federal government still classifies it as a Schedule I drug. That places Cannabis in the same category as heroin, officially considered to have no medical value and high potential for abuse. These claims have been disproven by decades of research and millions of patient experiences.

The contradiction is stark. In one state, adults can celebrate Cannabis openly, purchase it safely, and contribute tax revenue to their community. Cross an invisible line into another state, and that same action may result in fines, arrest, or imprisonment. This fractured system undermines the very idea of national unity and justice.

STATE VICTORIES AND MILESTONES

Colorado and Washington broke ground in 2012 as the first states to legalize adult use. Since then, the movement has swept the nation. California, Oregon, Nevada, Illinois, Michigan, New York, Massachusetts, Arizona, New Jersey, and dozens of others have joined the wave. By 2025, nearly half of all Americans live in states where recreational Cannabis is legal.

These victories transcend party lines. Voters in both conservative and progressive states have chosen freedom at the ballot box. The growing legalization map tells a story not of politics, but of people demanding a better way.

ECONOMIC AND SOCIAL BENEFITS

The benefits of legalization are not abstract. Recreational Cannabis has generated tens of billions in tax revenue, funding states' education system, healthcare, infrastructure, and community programs. It has created hundreds of thousands of jobs in cultivation, manufacturing, retail, technology, logistics, and tourism. Entire industries have emerged from what once was criminalized.

Legalization has also delivered profound social justice benefits. Arrests for Cannabis possession have plummeted, saving millions in law enforcement and court costs. Families once torn apart by nonviolent Cannabis charges are seeing relief. Communities disproportionately targeted by prohibition are beginning to benefit from expungement and equity programs. Cannabis legalization has proven to be not just an economic driver, but a tool for fairness and repair.

A SAFER CHOICE THAN ALCOHOL

Recreational Cannabis is not about promoting use. It is about giving adults safer choices. Unlike alcohol, Cannabis does not cause fatal poisonings, violent behavior, or long-term organ damage. Most adults who choose Cannabis describe relaxation, creativity, social connection, or rest.

This comparison highlights a lingering double standard. Alcohol is deeply embedded in American culture despite its well documented harms. Cannabis, safer by every measurable standard, remains stigmatized in many places.

The truth is clear: *responsible Cannabis use carries fewer risks and greater benefits than alcohol.*

THE ROAD AHEAD

The unfinished victory lies at the federal level. Until Cannabis is removed from Schedule I, businesses face banking restrictions, veterans are denied access through the VA, and interstate travel remains fraught with risk. Entrepreneurs, patients, and consumers continue to navigate uncertainty while waiting for Washington to catch up.

But momentum is undeniable. Every election cycle brings new states into the fold. Every year, more lawmakers cross the aisle to support reform. Courts, corporations, and communities alike are preparing for the inevitable; full national legalization. The question is no longer if it will happen, but when.

WHY THIS MATTERS

Recreational Cannabis matters because freedom matters. Adults deserve the right to make their own choices about what they consume, just as they do with alcohol or caffeine. Families deserve the safety of regulated markets rather than the risks of the illicit trade. Communities deserve the economic growth, tax revenue, and justice reforms that legalization provides.

This chapter is not just about Cannabis, it is about America growing up and admitting the failures of prohibition. It is about building a future that values science over fear, compassion over stigma, and freedom over punishment.

Recreational Cannabis is not just a product on a shelf. It is a symbol of victory, resilience, and progress. It marks the beginning of a new chapter in American life, one where choice, safety, and justice finally take precedence over fear, hypocrisy, and outdated laws.

BEYOND THE BASICS

"Beyond the basics, Cannabis becomes less about controversy and more about understanding how to use it responsibly, precisely, and with respect for the science that guides its future."

26

DELIVERY METHODS

EXPLORING THE OPTIONS

Cannabis is one plant, but there are countless ways to experience its benefits. Modern innovation has transformed a single flower into an entire spectrum of delivery methods. Each method offers its own rhythm, feel, and purpose. Some provide rapid relief, while others offer steady and long-lasting effects. Some emphasize ritual and tradition, while others focus on precision and convenience. What matters most is that adults today have the freedom to choose the approach that fits their lifestyle, health needs, or even the moment they are in.

FLOWER

The dried flower remains the classic and most widely recognized form of Cannabis. For generations it has been rolled into joints, packed into pipes, or shared through bongs. Flower delivers an immediate effect because cannabinoids and terpenes are inhaled directly into the lungs and absorbed into the bloodstream within moments. The full aroma and flavor profile of the plant is experienced most vividly through this form, which is why many enthusiasts consider flower the most authentic expression of Cannabis.

Today, vaporizing flower has become increasingly popular. Tabletop vaporizers and handheld devices heat Cannabis without burning it, releasing cannabinoids and terpenes as a clean vapor that preserves both taste and potency. This reduces exposure to smoke and makes the experience smoother while still providing rapid relief. Flower remains the foundation of Cannabis culture because it carries not only medicinal value but also tradition, ritual, and community.

EDIBLES

Edibles have quickly become one of the fastest growing categories in Cannabis. From gummies and chocolates to baked goods, savory snacks, and sparkling beverages, infused products offer a discreet, flavorful, and long-lasting experience. Unlike inhalation, which works within minutes, edibles take longer to activate because cannabinoids are absorbed through the digestive system and metabolized by the liver. Onset typically begins within thirty to ninety minutes, but the effects can last four to eight hours or longer.

This extended duration makes edibles particularly helpful for patients managing chronic conditions such as pain, insomnia, or nausea, where continuous relief is essential. Recreational consumers also favor edibles when they want a slow building, immersive experience. Advances in technology have made dosing more precise than ever, giving consumers confidence in knowing exactly what to expect.

TINCTURES AND OILS

Tinctures and oils offer one of the most versatile delivery methods. A few drops placed under the tongue allow cannabinoids to absorb quickly through the mucous membranes, producing effects within fifteen to forty-five minutes. The same drops can also be added to food or beverages for a slower onset and longer duration.

For patients, tinctures provide precision and consistency, making it easy to fine-tune dosing throughout the day. For adults seeking convenience, tinctures are discreet and portable, fitting easily into pockets or purses. They represent an intersection of medicine and lifestyle, offering both control and flexibility. A single dropper bottle can serve as both a therapeutic tool and a simple way to maintain balance and calm.

VAPE CARTRIDGES AND PENS

Vape cartridges and pens have revolutionized Cannabis use by making it discreet, fast, and easy. These devices heat concentrated Cannabis oil and deliver smooth inhalation with minimal odor. For people who want rapid relief without the lingering smell of smoke, vape pens provide an accessible option.

Formulations vary widely, ranging from high THC oils to balanced CBD blends, as well as strain-specific extracts that preserve the terpene profiles of classic cultivars. The portability of vape pens has made them especially popular with adults who need quick relief on the go. While quality and safety standards vary, regulated markets have introduced rigorous testing to ensure consumers know exactly what they are putting in their bodies.

TOPICALS

Cannabis infused creams, balms, and salves offer localized relief without intoxication. Applied directly to the skin, these products deliver cannabinoids to receptors in the skin, muscles, and nerves without entering the bloodstream in significant amounts. Topicals are widely used for soreness, inflammation, joint pain, and skin conditions such as eczema or psoriasis.

For athletes, topicals provide recovery support after strenuous workouts. For patients with arthritis or chronic pain, they bring targeted comfort that allows movement without systemic effects. From soothing lotions to cooling gels, topicals are one of the most approachable ways for newcomers to explore Cannabis. They embody the plant's potential as both a medicine and a wellness tool.

CAPSULES AND TABLETS

Capsules and tablets bring Cannabis into a format that feels familiar to anyone who takes traditional medicine. Each dose is pre-measured and consistent, making it easy to integrate into daily routines. Onset typically occurs within thirty to sixty minutes, with effects lasting four to six hours.

This method is especially valuable for patients managing long-term conditions who need steady, predictable relief without the variability of inhalation or edibles. Capsules allow Cannabis to be taken discreetly alongside other medications, and they are increasingly favored in clinical settings for their precision and standardization.

ONSET AND DURATION AT A GLANCE

Each delivery method has its own rhythm.

Flower and vapes: *effects begin within minutes and last one to three hours.*

Edibles: *begin within thirty to ninety minutes and last four to eight hours.*

Tinctures and oils: *begin within fifteen to forty-five minutes and last two to four hours.*

Capsules and tablets: *begin within thirty to sixty minutes and last four to six hours.*

Topicals: *provide localized effects within minutes, lasting one to three hours.*

This variety allows adults to tailor Cannabis use to their needs, whether they seek quick relief, long lasting calm, or targeted comfort.

A WORLD OF CHOICE

The true power of modern Cannabis lies not only in its effectiveness but in its flexibility.

Adults can choose the method that suits their needs: *the ritual of flower, the creativity of edibles, the precision of tinctures, the convenience of vape pens, the familiarity of capsules, or the gentleness of topicals.*

Each delivery method represents innovation and progress, expanding the ways Cannabis can be safely and effectively integrated into daily life.

WHY THIS MATTERS

Delivery methods matter because they turn Cannabis from an abstract idea into a personal and practical experience. They allow individuals to decide not just whether to use Cannabis, but how to use it. They make Cannabis adaptable, to lifestyles, to health needs, to moments of celebration, and to moments of healing.

This is not about one plant fitting into one box. Cannabis is a spectrum of possibilities. It is a tool as diverse as the people who use it. Every method is another door opened, another opportunity for balance, relief, and joy.

Cannabis is not one experience but a spectrum of possibilities, shaped by choice, intention, and the way it is delivered.

27

TERPENES AND THE ENTOURAGE EFFECT

THE LANGUAGE OF AROMAS

Every time you open a jar of Cannabis, the first thing you notice is the aroma. Some strains smell citrusy and bright, others earthy and grounding, and others sweet or even spicy. These scents come from terpenes, natural compounds found in Cannabis.

Terpenes do more than create fragrances. They help guide how Cannabis feels when it is used.

Limonene, also found in lemons, brings uplifting and mood-brightening qualities. Myrcene, common in mangos and hops, promotes calm and relaxation. Pinene, from pine trees, adds clarity and focus.

Together, terpenes form each strain's fingerprint, shaping its personality and influencing the experience in ways that cannabinoids alone cannot.

THE SCIENCE OF THE ENTOURAGE EFFECT

For decades, Cannabis research was focused on single compounds such as THC. Pharmaceutical companies even produced synthetic THC, known as Marinol, to treat nausea and loss of appetite. Yet patients often found the experience flat and unpleasant. Relief felt incomplete, and side effects like anxiety or dizziness were common.

By contrast, whole-plant Cannabis felt balanced and more therapeutic.

This observation led scientists to the concept of the entourage effect: *the idea that cannabinoids, terpenes, and other plant compounds work together in harmony, amplifying benefits while softening side effects.*

Science has since confirmed what patients knew. CBD tempers THC's intensity, easing anxiety while extending relief. Myrcene appears to increase cell permeability, allowing cannabinoids to act more efficiently. Limonene and pinene add uplifting or focusing qualities, reshaping how the core cannabinoids are experienced.

Because of this interplay, two strains with the same THC percentage can feel entirely different. One may bring restlessness while another promotes calm. The difference lies in its supporting cast of terpenes and minor cannabinoids working together as one.

A BRIDGE BETWEEN SCIENCE AND EXPERIENCE

The beauty of the entourage effect is that it connects measurable science with human experience. When patients describe one strain as creative and another as relaxing, they are describing chemistry in motion. Each terpene and cannabinoid acts like an instrument, subtle on its own but transformative together.

Researchers are now mapping these interactions. Early studies show that certain combinations of terpenes and cannabinoids may influence specific pathways related to mood, inflammation, or neuroprotection. What once sounded like anecdote is becoming measurable biology. The result is a new language that turns personal testimony into data and data into understanding.

PRACTICAL APPLICATIONS

The entourage effect has practical value for both patients and consumers.

A person managing chronic pain may choose a strain rich in THC balanced with myrcene and linalool to promote relaxation and sleep. Someone with depression may find greater benefit from a lower-THC strain with limonene, which helps elevate mood.

Individuals sensitive to THC often prefer CBD-dominant profiles that reduce psychoactive intensity while still providing comfort.

For these reasons, broad-spectrum and full-spectrum products often perform better than isolates. Nature designed Cannabis as a complete plant, and its compounds appear to function best when left together rather than separated.

A NOTE ON TERPENE VARIETY

Cannabis contains a remarkably wide range of terpenes, well over one hundred have been identified across different strains. Various publications list six, seven, or even more primary terpenes depending on concentration, frequency, and available research. For clarity and consistency, this book highlights the six terpenes most commonly found in modern cannabis and the ones most strongly supported by scientific literature. These core six provide a reliable foundation for understanding how aroma and therapeutic effects take shape, even though many additional terpenes contribute in smaller, strain specific ways.

MAJOR TERPENES AND THEIR EFFECTS

Myrcene: *Musky and earthy, found in mangos and hops. Associated with relaxation and rest.*

Limonene: *Citrus aroma, found in lemons and oranges. Uplifting, stress reducing, and mood enhancing.*

Pinene: *Fresh pine scent, found in rosemary and pine trees. Improves focus, alertness, and may support open airways.*

Linalool: *Floral and lavender like. Known for calming effects, easing anxiety, and supporting sleep.*

Caryophyllene: *Spicy and peppery, found in black pepper and cloves. Unique because it interacts with CB2 receptors, supporting inflammation relief.*

Humulene: *Woody and earthy, found in hops and coriander. Linked to focus and appetite regulation.*

Each terpene contributes its own voice, and together they create the plant's full character.

(See Appendix, Figure 4: Terpene Wheel)

TERPENES BEYOND CANNABIS

Terpenes are not exclusive to Cannabis. They are part of nature's design. The same compounds that calm or energize us in Cannabis also fill the natural world. Lavender fields, pine forests, and citrus groves all speak to us through terpenes.

This is why aromatherapy works through similar chemistry. The scent of pine clears the mind because of pinene. Lavender soothes because of linalool. Cannabis simply gathers many of these familiar plant effects into a single source, allowing people to experience nature's chemistry in one concentrated form. Seen this way, Cannabis is not an exception, it is an amplifier of what plants have been doing for millions of years.

WHY THIS MATTERS

Terpenes reveal the nuance of Cannabis. They explain why products with the same THC content can deliver completely different results. They remind us that healing comes from balance rather than intensity.

The entourage effect shifts the focus from potency to composition. It teaches that the magic of Cannabis lies not in a single molecule but in the relationships among many. For patients, this means relief that is smoother and more tailored. For researchers, it offers a framework for designing more precise therapies.

Cannabis is more than a number on a label; it is a living collaboration of cannabinoids, terpenes, and plant compounds working together with the body. To overlook the entourage effect is to overlook the essence of what makes this plant extraordinary.

EMERGING RESEARCH AND FUTURE POTENTIAL

Scientists are only beginning to explore how deep this synergy runs. Some are studying terpene ratios to guide specific outcomes such as focus, calm, or sleep. Others are examining how terpenes act as natural biomodulators, helping cannabinoids cross cellular barriers or influence brain signaling.

Future formulations may combine terpenes in the same way nutritionists balance vitamins or amino acids, each element supporting the others. As this research expands, understanding terpenes will become as essential to Cannabis science as understanding cannabinoids themselves.

The entourage effect is more than a scientific theory. It is proof that nature's design is already intelligent. Every aroma, every molecule, every subtle shift in mood is part of a complex harmony that we are only beginning to understand.

28

THE FUTURE OF CANNABIS MEDICINE

A GLOBAL FRONTIER

Around the world, Cannabis research is accelerating at a pace that would have seemed impossible only a decade ago. In Israel, researchers have spent more than forty years studying the plant, producing hundreds of peer reviewed papers and clinical trials that make the country a global leader in Cannabis science. Canada has not only legalized Cannabis nationally but has woven it into its healthcare system, where doctors prescribe it for conditions ranging from chronic pain to post traumatic stress disorder. Germany recently voted in favor of full legalization, creating one of the largest regulated Cannabis markets in Europe. Australia, the United Kingdom, and countries across Africa and South America are all moving forward with structured programs for both research and patient access.

The global trend is undeniable. Cannabis is no longer dismissed as fringe or counterculture. It is being embraced as a mainstream tool of modern medicine and wellness. The question is not if Cannabis will define the next frontier of medicine, but how quickly nations will act to embrace it, and who will lead, and who will be left behind.

INNOVATION ON THE HORIZON

The Cannabis of tomorrow will look very different from the Cannabis of today. For much of the twentieth century, Cannabis was viewed through a narrow lens, mostly as a single compound, THC. Today, researchers are looking far beyond THC and CBD to a spectrum of more than one hundred minor cannabinoids, each with its own therapeutic promise.

Researchers are now studying an expanding list of lesser known cannabinoids, each with unique therapeutic potential.

CBG: *showing potential for inflammation, gut health, and antibacterial effects.*

CBN: *studied for sleep and neuroprotection.*

THCV: *linked to appetite regulation and glucose control.*

At the same time, terpene profiling has advanced to the point where blends can be designed with remarkable precision. Imagine a formula crafted specifically for restorative sleep that combines CBD, CBN, and linalool, or one designed for focus and productivity with THCV, pinene, and limonene. Doctors are beginning to view Cannabis not as one plant, but as an entire customizable toolkit.

Technological breakthroughs are adding even more possibilities. Nanotechnology is being used to increase absorption rates and predict onset times with precision. Smart inhalers and dose controlled vaporizers allow patients to receive the exact amount they need, monitored and recorded digitally. Topical patches deliver steady doses over twelve or twenty-four hours. The future of Cannabis medicine is not a joint passed between friends, it is a tailored prescription crafted for an individual's biology, delivered with scientific accuracy.

THE UNCERTAIN AMERICAN PATH

While much of the world moves forward, the United States remains mired in contradiction. At the federal level, Cannabis is still classified as a Schedule I drug, the most restrictive category, shared with heroin. Under this classification, Cannabis is considered to have *"no medical use"* and a *"high potential for abuse."* These claims have been disproven by decades of science and millions of patients.

The contradiction grows sharper when compared to other substances. Fentanyl, a synthetic opioid responsible for tens of thousands of overdose deaths each year, is scheduled lower than Cannabis. Alcohol, which kills more than one hundred forty-thousand Americans annually, is fully legal. Cannabis, safer by every measure, remains criminalized at the federal level.

This classification creates ripple effects that punish everyone. Researchers struggle to obtain approval to study Cannabis. Doctors are restricted from recommending it. Patients are denied safe and reliable access. Businesses are shut out of basic banking services. Veterans cannot receive Cannabis through the VA, even if their doctors believe it would help. Families in states without reform are left to suffer while their neighbors across state lines live with freedom and choice.

Each year of delay means more preventable deaths, more suffering, and more lives diminished by stigma and politics.

THE POLITICS OF RESISTANCE

Some states have gone beyond delay to outright regression. Texas stands as a prime example. As mentioned in Chapter 21, Texas Lieutenant Governor Dan Patrick has consistently blocked expansion of the state's limited medical program and now supports efforts to ban all forms of THC, including hemp derived cannabinoids that are federally legal. These moves are not about protecting families. They are about protecting political power.

Other states, including Idaho, Kansas, and Nebraska, remain entrenched in prohibition, refusing even the most basic reforms. For families living in these places, the injustice is particularly painful. Parents must uproot their lives and move across state lines to obtain treatment for sick children. Veterans must choose between suffering or breaking the law. Meanwhile, leaders in these states continue to defend outdated laws that harm rather than protect.

PROJECTIONS AND POSSIBILITIES

Despite resistance, the momentum for Cannabis is unstoppable. Analysts predict that the global Cannabis market could exceed one hundred billion dollars within the next decade. That projection does not simply represent economic opportunity. It represents millions of patients whose lives could be improved.

Cannabis is being studied for conditions that stretch across nearly every field of medicine: *pain, anxiety, depression, epilepsy, cancer care,* *sleep disorders, neurodegenerative diseases, autoimmune conditions, metabolic disorders, and more.*

The future will not treat Cannabis as a one size fits all plant but as a suite of therapeutic tools integrated into standard healthcare.

But progress is not guaranteed. Federal legalization in the United States has stalled repeatedly. Lobbyists from the alcohol, pharmaceutical, and private prison industries continue to fight reform, pouring millions into campaigns designed to protect their interests. The future of Cannabis medicine will require persistence from patients, doctors, advocates, and voters who demand better.

WHY THIS MATTERS

The future of Cannabis medicine matters because it is about more than a plant. It is about whether science will be allowed to guide policy, or whether politics and profit will continue to dictate healthcare. It is about whether families will have access to safe options, or whether they will be forced into suffering because of outdated laws.

This matters for patients. Children with epilepsy deserve medicine that stops their seizures. Veterans with PTSD deserve sleep without nightmares. Cancer patients deserve relief from pain and nausea. None of these should be controversial.

This matters for science. Researchers deserve the freedom to explore the full potential of Cannabis without political handcuffs. Doctors deserve the ability to recommend what works, not what is politically convenient.

This matters for freedom. Adults deserve the right to make their own choices about their health and wellbeing. Communities deserve the economic growth, tax revenue, and justice reform that come with legalization.

History will remember the politicians who delayed Cannabis reform as those who chose ideology over evidence and profit over people. They will not be remembered as visionaries, but as obstacles who allowed their citizens to suffer. Leaders like Dan Patrick may succeed in slowing progress, but they cannot stop it.

The future belongs to truth, and the truth is that Cannabis helps people. The only question is whether America will seize this future or fall behind as other nations lead the way.

29

CONCLUSION (FROM REEFER MADNESS TO REALITY)

THE BIRTH OF A LIE

In 1937, Harry Anslinger, the first commissioner of the Federal Bureau of Narcotics, stood before Congress and declared: *"Marijuana is the most violence causing drug in the history of mankind."*

Those words were not science. They were theater. They became the script for the propaganda film *Reefer Madness* and the foundation for a national hysteria that would last for generations.

Anslinger's campaign was not designed to protect health. It was driven by politics, prejudice, and control. He exploited racism, fanned fear, and used Cannabis as a weapon to expand his power. His words lit the match for an era in which a plant that had been used as medicine for centuries was suddenly painted as a menace.

What followed was not protection but persecution. Prohibition policies jailed patients, silenced doctors, and erased centuries of healing knowledge. *Reefer Madness* was never just a movie. It was a warning of what happens when governments build policy on lies.

THE TRUTH EMERGES

Eighty years later, the smoke has cleared and the truth stands unshaken. Cannabis is not the cause of violence, chaos, or decline. It is a source of relief, restoration, and balance.

Across these pages, we have witnessed Cannabis ease the suffering of people living with Alzheimer's, epilepsy, cancer, chronic pain, fibromyalgia, multiple sclerosis, Parkinson's, arthritis, Crohn's disease, glaucoma, migraines, diabetes, autism, and countless other conditions once thought untouchable by modern medicine.

We have seen it bring rest to children whose seizures once defined every moment of their lives. We have seen it restore dignity to veterans haunted by memories of war. We have seen it provide adults with a safer choice than alcohol, offering calm and connection instead of harm and despair.

We have explored delivery methods that turn Cannabis into a tool for daily living. We have studied terpenes and the entourage effect, which reveal that Cannabis is not just THC in isolation, but a symphony of compounds working in harmony with the body.

Science now confirms what patients have known all along: *the whole plant offers more than the sum of its parts.*

The truth is not complicated. Cannabis helps people. It is not the menace Harry Anslinger described in 1937. It is medicine. It is wellness. It is dignity, compassion, and hope made tangible.

SCIENCE OVER STIGMA

For decades, research was blocked, distorted, or outright banned. Yet even under these constraints, scientists uncovered remarkable truths.

The discovery of the Endocannabinoid System revealed that the human body is designed to work in partnership with cannabinoids. This natural system regulates sleep, appetite, mood, memory, pain, and immunity. Cannabis does not invade the body. It harmonizes with it.

International research continues to confirm this partnership. In Israel, clinical trials demonstrate Cannabis reducing seizures, calming autism symptoms, and improving quality of life. In Canada, Cannabis is integrated into the national healthcare system, prescribed openly for chronic pain, PTSD, and cancer care. In Europe, doctors prescribe Cannabis alongside conventional medicines, while universities fund studies into neurodegenerative disease and immune disorders.

The science is clear. The only question is whether society has the courage to act on it.

THE AMERICAN CONTRADICTION

Nowhere is the divide sharper than in the United States. Some states embrace Cannabis, building thriving medical and recreational markets, generating billions in tax revenue, reducing arrests, and expanding patient access. Others cling to prohibition, leaving families desperate, veterans unsupported, and patients criminalized.

In Texas, elected leaders vocally push to ban even hemp derived cannabinoids, ignoring evidence and silencing patients. Meanwhile, in Colorado, California, and New York, Americans walk into dispensaries with the freedom to purchase safely tested Cannabis products.

This contradiction undermines science, compassion, and justice. It is the last echo of *Reefer Madness* reverberating through modern policy.

THE HUMAN COST

Behind every statistic is a story, and behind every story is a life. A veteran who finally sleeps through the night without nightmares. A child whose seizures stop after years of torment. A grandmother who finds enough relief from arthritis to hold her grandchildren without wincing. A cancer patient who regains the appetite and strength to endure treatment with dignity. A Parkinson's patient who steadies their tremors long enough to sign their own name again.

Cannabis is not an abstract issue or a political talking point. It is lived reality. These are not numbers in a report or figures on a graph. They are families rediscovering hope, parents reclaiming joy, and patients finding comfort in bodies that had only known pain.

The cost of delay is not measured in policies or votes. It is measured in lost days, in unnecessary suffering, and in lives diminished when relief was already within reach. Every year of prohibition has meant more nights without sleep, more meals pushed away in nausea, and more families forced to watch loved ones endure pain that could have been eased.

The human cost of prohibition is not theoretical. It is immediate, it is ongoing, and it is preventable. This cost, paid every day by ordinary people, makes the case for change undeniable.

A GLOBAL MOVEMENT

The world is moving forward. Israel integrates Cannabis into hospital systems. Canada provides it through national healthcare. Germany, Malta, and other European nations are opening regulated markets. Australia is expanding access for patients and building a medical export economy. Nations across Africa and South America are exploring Cannabis as both medicine and opportunity.

Projections estimate the global Cannabis industry could surpass one hundred billion dollars in the next decade. But the real number that matters is not market size. It is the millions of lives improved by access to safe, regulated Cannabis.

The United States faces a choice: *will it lead this movement or continue to lag behind, tied to the ghost of Anslinger's lies?*

THE FAILURE OF AMERICAN LEADERSHIP

The greatest tragedy of Cannabis prohibition is not ignorance. It is willful failure. For nearly a century, American leaders have had access to the science, the stories, and the truth. And yet, again and again, they have chosen politics over people.

In Washington, lawmakers sit in air conditioned offices guarded by police and protected by privilege. Their greatest risks are losing votes or missing reelection. Meanwhile, the very veterans who fought to protect those offices live with nightmares, broken bodies, and untreated trauma. Parents watch their children seize in hospital beds while safe treatments are locked away by federal laws. Patients with cancer, chronic pain, and degenerative diseases are left to suffer while politicians debate semantics.

Other nations have moved forward. Israel funds clinical research. Canada provides Cannabis through national healthcare. Germany, Europe, and Australia regulate markets that balance access and safety. Even emerging nations across Africa and South America are embracing Cannabis as medicine and opportunity.

And yet the United States, the wealthiest, most powerful nation on earth, clings to a lie born in 1937. Leaders who claim to *"support the troops"* deny veterans Cannabis through the VA. Leaders who speak of *"protecting children"* deny parents the medicine that stops seizures. Leaders who campaign on *"freedom"* criminalize adults for making a safer choice than alcohol.

This is not just neglect. It is betrayal. It is the United States government failing its own people, generation after generation.

But history is moving. The truth is out. The people know what their leaders refuse to admit. That reality is the foundation of the next fight, the fight between a government built on prohibition and the citizens demanding freedom.

This is where the next story begins.

WHY THIS MATTERS

This book began with history. It moved through science, told stories, celebrated victories, and confronted injustice. It was written for patients seeking relief, for parents searching for hope, for veterans demanding dignity, for doctors pursuing evidence, and for readers who simply wanted the truth.

Cannabis is more than a plant. It is a mirror reflecting what kind of society we choose to be. One ruled by fear and politics, or one guided by science, compassion, and courage.

It matters because children are still seizing in hospital beds while medicine sits locked behind laws. It matters because veterans who risked their lives for freedom return home only to be denied the very medicine that helps them survive. It matters because families are still uprooting their lives, crossing borders, or risking arrest just to care for those they love.

It matters because prohibition has never been equal. Communities of color and the poor have borne the brunt of arrests, convictions, and incarceration. Thousands still carry criminal records for a plant that is now sold legally in polished dispensaries. Justice demands that legalization include repair, equity, and opportunity.

It matters because delay costs lives, health, and dignity. America spends billions on prisons and drug wars while refusing to invest in research, healthcare, and healing. Other nations move forward. America clings to a lie born in 1937.

And it matters because Cannabis is not just about today. It is about the future. The future of medicine, the future of wellness, the future of justice, and the future of freedom.

FROM REEFER MADNESS TO REALITY

The conclusion is undeniable. Cannabis belongs in medicine, in wellness, and in society. It belongs in the doctor's toolkit, the caregiver's hand, and the patient's life. To deny it is to deny science, compassion, and common sense.

History is watching. Generations ahead will ask whether we had the courage to clear the smoke and see reality for what it is. The time is now.

Cannabis matters because people matter. Every life eased, every family healed, every injustice undone is proof that truth is stronger than fear. To do less is not caution; it is cruelty disguised as policy!

Cannabis matters because people matter, and any society that denies healing in the face of truth is choosing fear over humanity.

APPENDIX

The following figures provide visual reference for key biological systems and concepts discussed throughout the book, including the Endocannabinoid System, cannabinoid receptor distribution, clinical endocannabinoid deficiency, and terpene profiles.

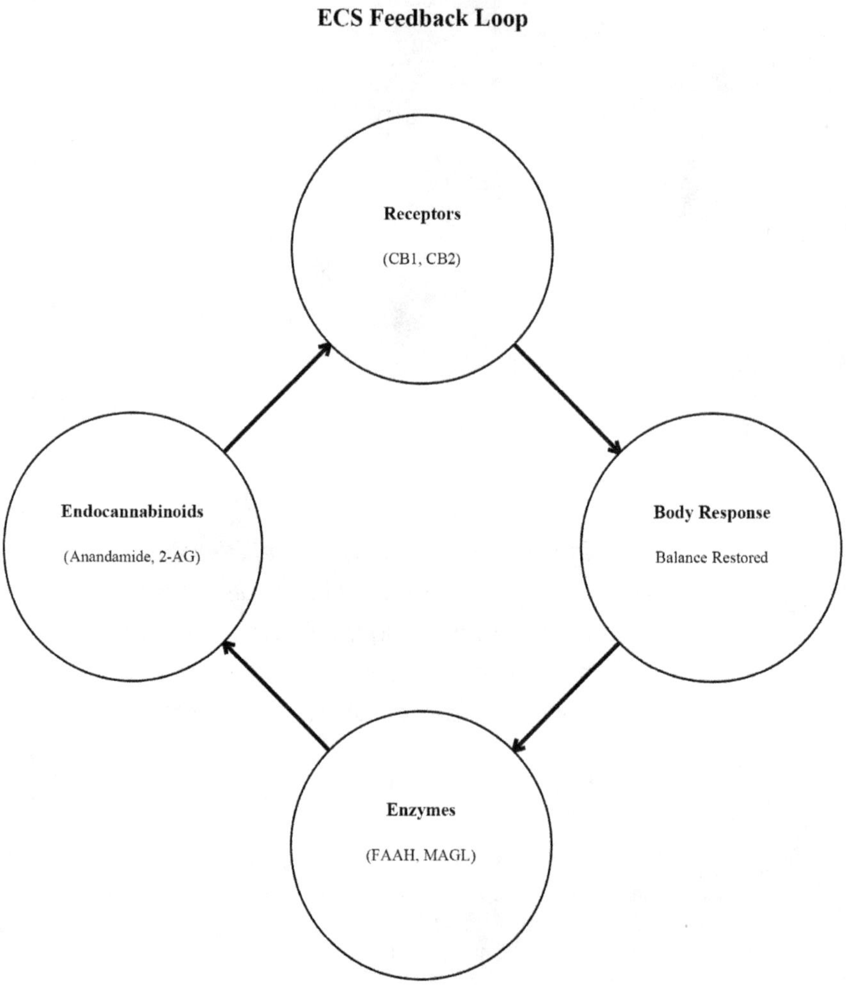

Figure 1: Endocannabinoid System *(ESC Feedback Loop)*

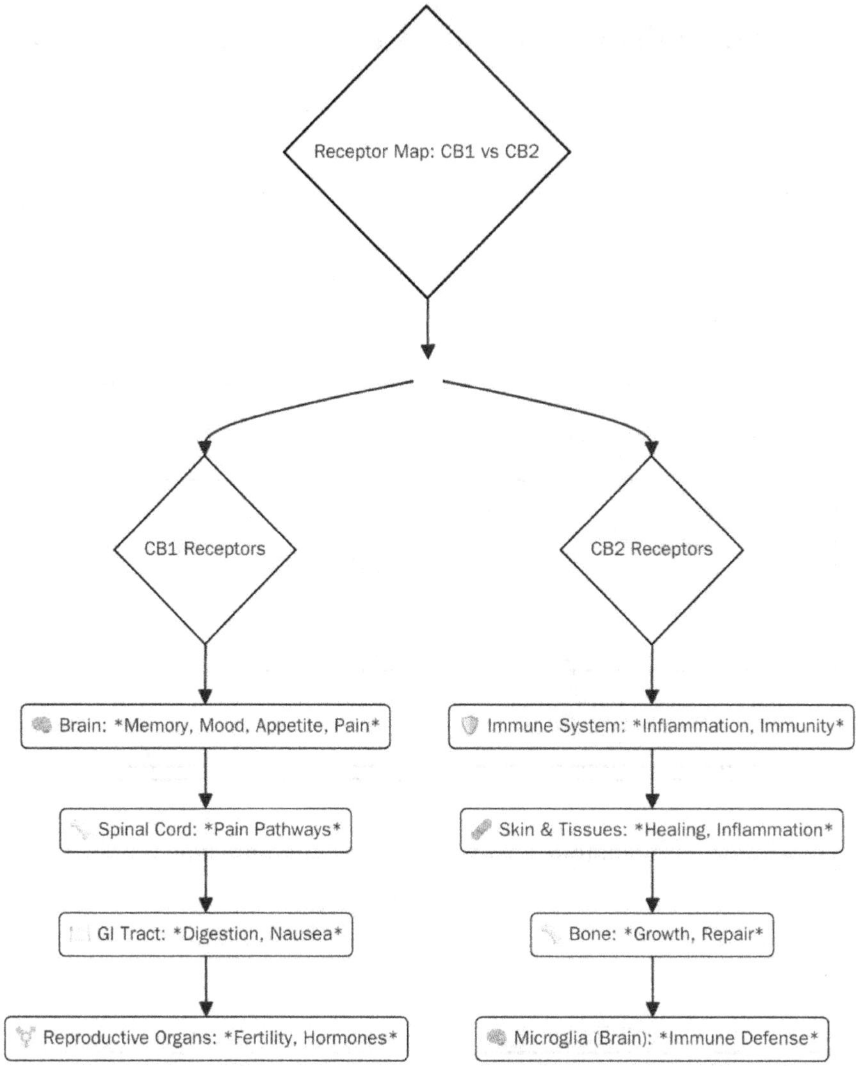

Figure 2: Receptor Map

Clinical Endocannabinoid Deficiency (CECD) Flow

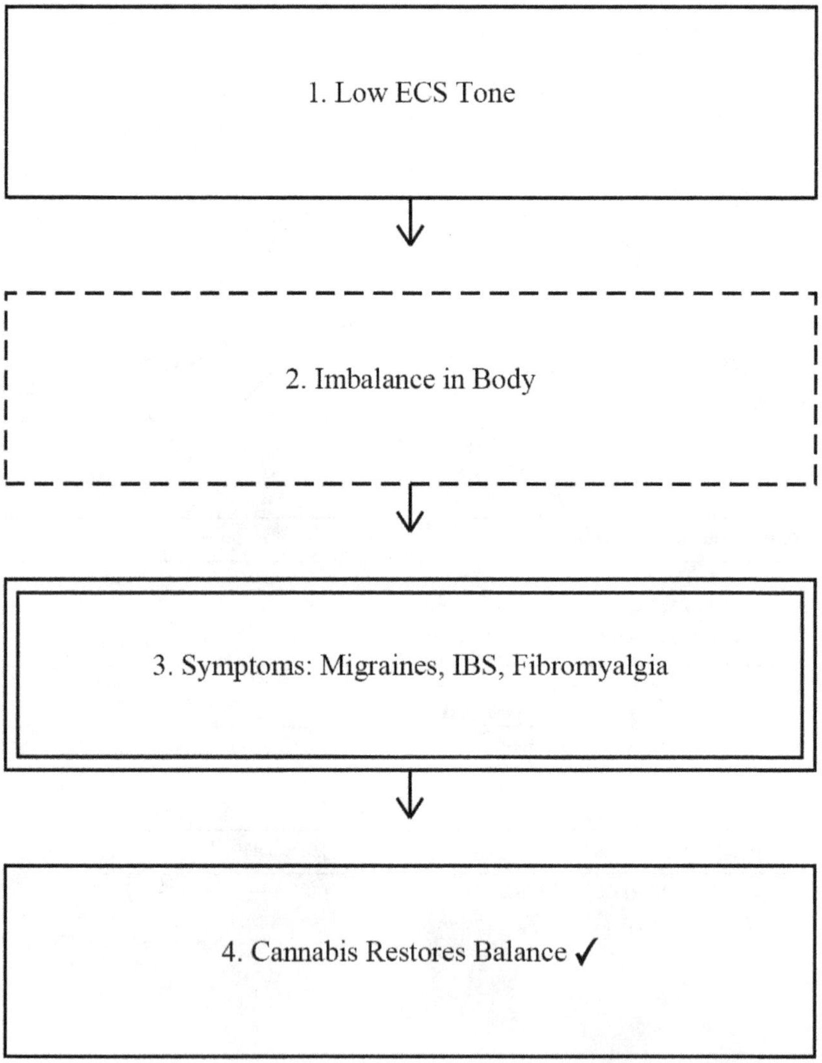

Figure 3: Clinical Endocannabinoid Deficiency (*CECD*) Flow

Terpene Wheel: Aromas and Effects

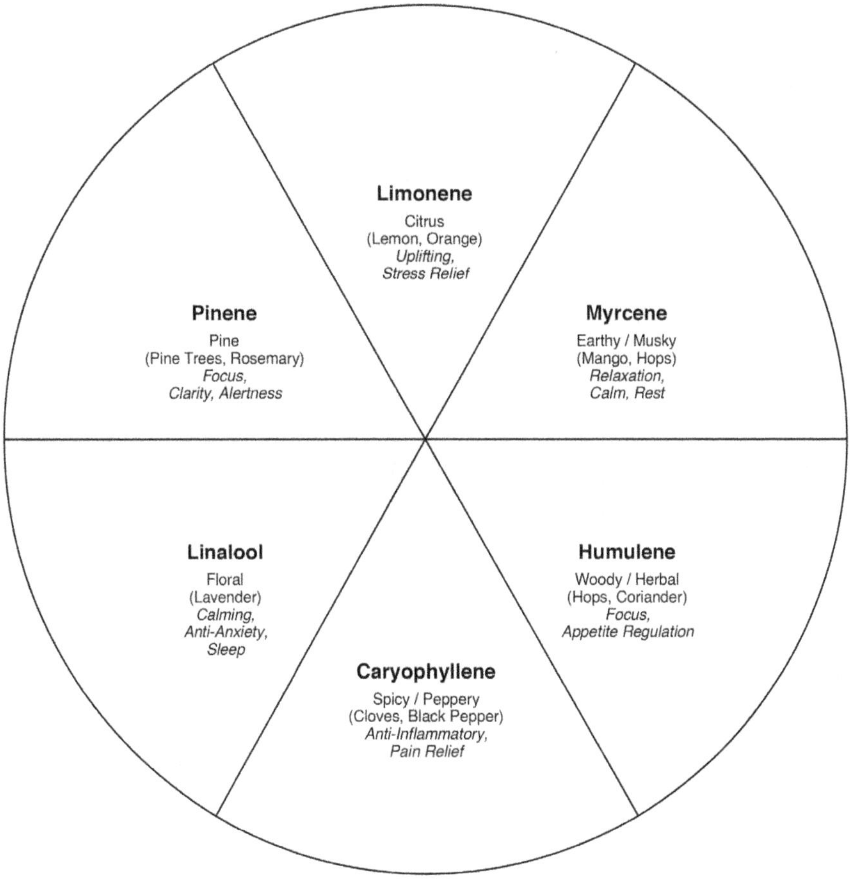

Figure 4: Terpene Wheel (*Aromas and Effect*)

GLOSSARY

A

2-AG - One of the body's two main endocannabinoids that activates cannabinoid receptors to maintain balance.

Adenosine Signaling *(ad-uh-noh-seen)* - A biochemical process that helps calm the nervous system and reduce seizure activity.

Alzheimer's Disease *(alts-hy-merz)* - A neurodegenerative disorder causing memory loss and cognitive decline; cannabis may reduce inflammation and improve quality of life.

Amyloid Beta *(am-uh-loid)* - A protein fragment that accumulates in the brain in Alzheimer's, contributing to neurodegeneration.

Anandamide *(uh-nan-duh-mide)* - A natural endocannabinoid known as the "bliss molecule," supporting mood and balance.

Anxiolytic *(ang-zee-oh-lit-ik)* - A substance that reduces anxiety and promotes calm; many cannabinoids and terpenes, such as CBD and linalool, have anxiolytic properties.

Appetite Regulation - The process by which the body manages hunger and satiety; influenced by CB1 receptors.

Arachidonoylglycerol *(uh-rack-ih-don-oyl-gliss-er-ol)* - The full biochemical name for 2-AG, a major endocannabinoid synthesized from arachidonic acid that works alongside anandamide to activate CB1 and CB2 receptors.

Autoimmune Disease *(aw-toe-ih-myoon)* - A condition where the immune system attacks healthy tissue; cannabis helps regulate this response.

B

Basal Ganglia - A group of brain structures controlling movement and coordination; affected in Parkinson's disease and influenced by CB1 receptors.

Beta-Caryophyllene *(bay-tuh care-ee-off-uh-leen)* - A terpene that binds to CB2 receptors, reducing inflammation and pain.

Beta Cell Function - The insulin-producing cells of the pancreas; improved by THCV in studies of type 2 diabetes.

Beta-Endorphins - Natural opioid-like compounds produced by the brain that reduce pain and elevate mood.

Blood–Brain Barrier - A membrane protecting the brain from harmful substances while allowing nutrients and select compounds through.

Bone Remodeling - The continuous cycle of bone breakdown and rebuilding; influenced by CB2 receptor activity.

C

Cachexia *(ka-kek-see-uh)* - Muscle and weight loss caused by chronic illness; often improved by THC.

Cannabichromene ***(CBC)*** *(kan-uh-bih-kroh-meen)* - A minor cannabinoid with anti-inflammatory and neuroprotective properties.

Cannabidiol ***(CBD)*** *(kan-uh-bid-eye-ol)* - A non-intoxicating cannabinoid known for reducing anxiety, inflammation, and seizures.

Cannabidiolic Acid ***(CBDA)*** (kan-uh-bid-eye-ol-ik) - The raw precursor of CBD with strong anti-nausea and anti-seizure potential.

Cannabigerol ***(CBG)*** (kan-uh-bij-er-all) - A cannabinoid that supports focus, gut health, and neuroprotection.

Cannabinol *(CBN)* (kan-uh-bin-ahl) - A mildly psychoactive cannabinoid that forms as THC oxidizes, promoting sleep.

Cannabis - A plant genus containing psychoactive and

non-psychoactive compounds used for therapeutic purposes.

Cannabinoid Receptors *(CB1, CB2)* - Specialized cell receptors that interact with cannabinoids to regulate mood, pain, and immune response.

Cannabinoids (kuh-nab-ih-noydz) - Active compounds in cannabis such as THC, CBD, and CBG.

CB1 Receptor - Found in the brain and nervous system; responsible for regulating coordination, mood, and memory.

CB2 Receptor - Found primarily in immune and peripheral tissues; reduces inflammation and supports immune balance.

CECD *(Clinical Endocannabinoid Deficiency)* - The theory that low endocannabinoid levels contribute to chronic conditions such as migraines and fibromyalgia.

Chemotherapy-Induced Nausea and Vomiting *(CINV)* - A side effect of cancer-treatment effectively reduced by THC.

Chronic Pain - Persistent pain lasting over three months; a leading reason for medical cannabis use.

Ciliary Body *(sil-ee-air-ee)* - The part of the eye that controls fluid drainage and pressure; affected by cannabinoids in glaucoma care.

Cognitive Decline - Gradual loss of mental ability linked to neurodegenerative disorders.

Crohn's Disease - A chronic inflammatory bowel disease that causes pain and digestive problems; cannabis reduces inflammation and restores appetite.

Cytokines *(sigh-toe-kines)* - Immune proteins that drive inflammation; cannabis helps regulate their release.

Cytokine Storm - An excessive immune response causing widespread inflammation and tissue damage; cannabinoids may help regulate this process in autoimmune and inflammatory diseases.

D

Dronabinol *(Marinol)* *(dro-nab-in-awl)* - A synthetic form of THC used medically for nausea and appetite loss.

Dravet Syndrome *(drah-vay)* - A severe form of childhood epilepsy effectively treated with CBD oil.

Dystonia *(dis-toe-nee-uh)* - Muscle contractions causing repetitive movements; improved by cannabis in certain neurological disorders.

E

ECS *(Endocannabinoid System)* - The body's biological network maintaining homeostasis across pain, mood, memory, and immunity.

Eczema *(Atopic Dermatitis)* *(ek-zuh-muh)* - A chronic inflammatory skin condition often soothed by CBD creams.

Endocannabinoids *(en-doh-kan-ab-ih-noydz)* - Molecules produced by the body that activate cannabinoid receptors to maintain balance.

Endothelium *(en-doh-thee-lee-um)* - The inner lining of blood vessels; cannabinoids promote relaxation through vasodilation.

Entourage Effect - The enhanced therapeutic synergy when cannabinoids and terpenes act together.

Epidiolex *(eh-pid-ee-oh-lecks)* - The first FDA-approved cannabis-derived medication for epilepsy.

Endocannabinoid Tone - The overall activity and health of the body's cannabinoid system.

Excitatory/Inhibitory Balance *(eksy-tuh-tore-ee)* - The brain's control between stimulation and calming signals; cannabinoids help restore this balance in epilepsy and autism.

Excitotoxicity *(ek-sy-toe-tok-sih-suh-tee)* - Damage to neurons caused by overstimulation; cannabinoids can protect against it.

F

FAAH ***(Fatty Acid Amide Hydrolase)*** - The enzyme that breaks down anandamide in the body.

Fibromyalgia *(fye-bro-my-al-juh)* - A chronic pain and fatigue disorder linked to endocannabinoid imbalance.

Frontotemporal Dementia - A degenerative brain disease involving personality and language changes; cannabis helps reduce agitation.

G

GABA ***(Gamma-Aminobutyric Acid)*** - A neurotransmitter that calms the brain; influenced by CBD.

GPR55 - A receptor modulated by CBD that helps regulate inflammation and brain activity.

Glaucoma - An eye disorder causing optic nerve damage; cannabis lowers intraocular pressure.

Glioblastoma *(gleeoh-blas-toe-muh)* - An aggressive brain cancer being studied for response to cannabinoids.

Gut–Brain Axis - The communication link between the digestive system and brain, balanced by endocannabinoid activity.

H

Hippocampus - A brain structure responsible for memory and learning, rich in CB1 receptors.

Homeostasis *(hoh-mee-oh-stay-sis)* - The body's natural state of balance regulated by the ECS.

Humulene *(hyoo-myoo-leen)* - A terpene with anti-inflammatory and appetite-suppressing effects.

Huntington's Disease - A neurodegenerative genetic condition; early data suggests neuroprotective benefits from cannabinoids.

Hypothalamus *(hi-puh-thal-uh-mus)* - A brain region controlling appetite, temperature, and stress responses; modulated by the ECS.

I

Immune Modulation - The balancing of immune system activity; cannabis reduces over-activation without full suppression.

Inflammation - The body's immune response to injury; chronic inflammation contributes to many diseases.

Insulin Resistance - The body's reduced ability to respond to insulin; cannabinoids may improve glucose control.

Ir**ritable Bowel Syndrome *(IBS)*** - A digestive disorder linked to stress and CECD; improved by CBD-rich formulations.

L

Lennox-Gastaut Syndrome *(len-ox gas-tow)* - A severe childhood epilepsy improved by cannabidiol treatment.

Limonene *(lim-oh-neen)* - A citrus terpene that uplifts mood and supports digestion.

Linalool *(lin-uh-lool)* - A lavender terpene with calming and

anti-anxiety effects.

Lupus - An autoimmune disease causing inflammation and pain; cannabis helps regulate immune overactivity.

M

MAGL *(Monoacylglycerol Lipase)* - The enzyme that breaks down the endocannabinoid 2-AG.

Migraines - Intense recurring headaches linked to CECD; cannabis reduces frequency and intensity.

Mood Regulation - Emotional stability maintained through balanced ECS signaling.

Multiple Sclerosis *(MS)* - An autoimmune disease damaging nerves; cannabis reduces spasticity, pain, and fatigue.

Myasthenia Gravis *(my-uhs-thee-nee-uh grav-is)* - A neuromuscular disorder; cannabinoids may improve fatigue and strength.

Myrcene *(meer-seen)* - A sedative terpene that enhances relaxation and sleep.

N

Nabiximols *(Sativex)* *(nah-bix-ih-mols)* - A pharmaceutical THC:CBD spray approved in several countries for MS spasticity.

Neurogenesis - The creation of new brain cells; cannabinoids may promote this in neurodegenerative diseases.

Neuroinflammation - Inflammation in the nervous system leading to disease; reduced by cannabinoids.

Neuropathic Pain - Nerve-based pain often improved by THC and CBD.

Neuroprotection - The preservation of nerve cells from damage through cannabinoid interaction.

Neurotransmitters - Brain chemicals that send messages between neurons, affected by cannabinoids.

O

Oromucosal *(or-oh-myoo-koh-suhl)* - Referring to administration through the mouth lining, as in nabiximols spray, for rapid absorption without smoking.

Osteoarthritis *(ahs-tee-oh-ar-thry-tis)* - A degenerative joint disease causing pain and stiffness; eased by cannabis.

Osteoporosis *(ahs-tee-oh-puh-roh-sis)* - A bone-weakening condition that may be slowed by CB2 activation.

Opioids - Strong painkillers with addiction risks; cannabis provides safer pain management.

Oxidative Stress - Cellular damage from free radicals; cannabinoids act as antioxidants.

P

Palliative Care *(palee-uh-tiv)* - Care focused on comfort in serious illness; cannabis enhances quality of life.

Parkinson's Disease *(par-kin-sunz)* - A neurodegenerative disorder causing tremors and rigidity; improved by cannabis therapy.

Peripheral Neuropathy - Nerve damage in hands or feet causing pain and numbness.

Phantom Limb Pain - Pain perceived in an amputated limb; cannabis reduces the sensation.

P**hotoreceptors** *(foh-toh-re-sep-turz)* - Light sensing cells in the retina; cannabinoids may help protect them from oxidative stress in glaucoma.

Pinene *(pie-neen)* - A terpene that supports focus, memory, and anti-inflammatory effects.

Post-Traumatic Stress Disorder *(PTSD)* - Trauma-related condition; cannabis calms fear circuits and improves sleep.

Psoriasis *(suh-rye-uh-sis)* - An autoimmune skin disease treated with cannabinoid topicals.

R

Receptors - Proteins on cell surfaces that receive and respond to cannabinoids and other molecules.

Retina - The light sensitive layer at the back of the eye that transmits visual signals to the brain; protected by cannabinoids.

Retinoid Receptors *(reh-tin-oyd ree-sep-turz)* - Proteins in skin and eye cells that regulate growth and repair; may interact with cannabinoids in inflammation control.

Rett Syndrome - A rare neurodevelopmental disorder where CBD shows potential benefits for seizures and behavior.

Reward Pathway - Brain system linked to pleasure and motivation, influenced by cannabinoids.

S

Sativex *(Nabiximols)* - THC-CBD spray used medically for MS related spasticity.

Serotonin - A neurotransmitter regulating mood and anxiety, influenced by CBD.

Sleep Regulation - A process controlled partly by the ECS; cannabinoids improve sleep onset and quality.

Spasticity - Muscle stiffness and spasms; cannabis helps relax muscles in MS and ALS.

Stress Response - The body's reaction to threat; cannabinoids lower cortisol and anxiety.

Sublingual - Refers to medications placed under the tongue for rapid absorption, common in cannabinoid oils and tinctures.

Sundowning - Evening agitation in dementia; improved with cannabis oils.

T

Tachyphylaxis *(tak-uh-fil-ak-sis)* - Diminished response to a drug after repeated use; relevant for dosing tolerance in long-term cannabis therapy.

Tetrahydrocannabinol *(THC)* (tet-ruh-hy-dro-kuh-nab-in-awl) The primary psychoactive compound in cannabis, providing pain relief and euphoria.

Tetrahydrocannabivarin *(THCV)*

(tet-ruh-hy-dro-kuh-nab-ih-vair-in) - A rare cannabinoid with potential to control appetite and blood sugar.

Terpenes - Aromatic compounds in cannabis that shape scent, flavor, and therapeutic effect.

Tourette's Syndrome - A neurological disorder causing tics; cannabis, especially THC, can reduce their frequency.

Transdermal *(trans-dur-muhl)* - Delivery of medicine through the skin into the bloodstream; used for cannabinoid patches and gels.

TRPV1 Channels - Pain and temperature sensors modulated by cannabinoids.

V

Vaporization - Heating cannabis to release cannabinoids without combustion, allowing fast relief.

Vasculature - The network of blood vessels; affected by THC's vasodilatory action improving circulation and intraocular pressure.

Vasodilation *(vay-so-die-lay-shun)* - The widening of blood vessels; THC promotes this to improve circulation.

W–Z

Whole-Plant Medicine - Using the full range of cannabinoids and terpenes for maximum therapeutic effect.

Withdrawal - Physical or psychological symptoms that occur after stopping certain drugs; cannabis can ease withdrawal from opioids or alcohol.

REFERENCES

American Glaucoma Society

Position Statement on Cannabis and Glaucoma. 2023

Since the 1970s, studies have shown THC can reduce intraocular pressure by up to 30%. The society continues to advocate for expanded research into long-term delivery methods and neuroprotective effects.

American Legion

National Survey on Veterans and Medical Cannabis. 2017

A landmark survey showing over 90% of veterans supported cannabis research and access through the VA system.

Anslinger, Harry J.

Testimony before the United States Congress on the Marihuana Tax Act. 1937

His testimony, filled with racist and sensational claims, set the foundation for federal prohibition.

Aran, Adi et al.

Cannabidiol-Rich Cannabis in Children with Autism Spectrum Disorder: Safety and Efficacy. Frontiers in Pharmacology, 2019

Evaluated CBD-rich preparations in children with severe behavioral challenges; caregivers reported improvements in behavior, communication, and anxiety.

Atharva Veda (Ayurvedic Text)

circa 2000 BCE

One of India's sacred Vedas references bhang as a sacred plant for anxiety, fever, and ceremony; an early medicinal cannabis record.

Avicenna, Ibn Sina

The Canon of Medicine. circa 1025 CE

A cornerstone of Islamic medical scholarship that described cannabis for pain and inflammation, influencing European pharmacopeias.

Basavarajappa, B. S.

"The Endocannabinoid System and Alzheimer's Disease." Neurochemistry International, 2017

Discussed ECS dysregulation in Alzheimer's and how cannabinoids may influence amyloid and tau pathologies.

Beta-Caryophyllene, Linalool, Myrcene, Pinene, Limonene, Humulene.
Various sources (2017–2024)
Primary terpenes documented for anti-inflammatory, analgesic, and neuroprotective activities across pharmacology literature.

Centers for Disease Control and Prevention (CDC)
Alcohol and Public Health: Data and Statistics. 2024
Provides national public health context and comparative epidemiology for substance use and policy.

Charlotte Figi
2012
Her extraordinary seizure reduction using CBD oil galvanized global attention, leading to the founding of nonprofit advocacy organizations and the path to FDA approval of Epidiolex.

Declaration of Independence
United States, 1776.
Early drafts were purportedly written on hemp paper, symbolizing hemp's historical role in early American industry.

Dennis Peron
California Proposition 215 (1996)
Activist and co-author of the first U.S. state medical cannabis legalization; credited with launching the modern movement.

Devinsky, Orrin et al.
"Trial of Cannabidiol for Drug-Resistant Seizures in the Dravet Syndrome." The New England Journal of Medicine, 2017
Randomized, placebo-controlled trial that showed CBD significantly reduced seizure frequency in children with Dravet syndrome.

Djaldetti, Ruth
"Cannabis in Parkinson's Disease: Clinical Experience." Tel Aviv University Medical Reports, 2014
Reported marked improvement in tremor, rigidity, sleep, and pain in Parkinson's patients following cannabis therapy.

Dr. Ethan Russo
"Clinical Endocannabinoid Deficiency: Toward Restoring Internal Balance." Neuro Endocrinology Letters, 2004
Proposed that conditions like migraine, fibromyalgia, and IBS may stem from low endocannabinoid tone; a conceptual framework for cannabinoid therapies.

Dr. Ethan Russo
"Taming THC: Potential Cannabis Synergy and Phytocannabinoid-Terpenoid Entourage Effects." British Journal of Pharmacology, 2011
Described how cannabinoids and terpenes interact synergistically to modulate physiological effects beyond any single compound.

Dr. Raphael Mechoulam
Hebrew University of Jerusalem, 1964 onward
Israeli chemist who isolated THC and helped reveal the Endocannabinoid System's functional role; his discoveries underpin modern cannabis science.

Dr. William C. Woodward (AMA)
Testimony before U.S. Congress opposing the Marihuana Tax Act 1937
As AMA delegate, he opposed Anslinger's prohibition narrative and advocated for cannabis's legitimate medical uses.

Ehrlichman, John
Interview by Dan Baum. Harper's Magazine, April 1994
A Nixon advisor admitted the "War on Drugs" was politically motivated to suppress Black and anti-war communities.

Epidiolex
FDA Approval, 2018
The first cannabis-derived drug approved by the U.S. FDA for Dravet and Lennox-Gastaut syndromes, validating decades of advocacy and clinical research.

Fitzcharles, Mary-Ann et al.
"Efficacy and Safety of Medical Cannabis in Chronic Pain and Rheumatic Conditions." Arthritis Care & Research, 2016
Systematic review showing meaningful pain and functional improvements in rheumatic disease patients using cannabis formulations.

Food and Drug Administration (U.S.)
"FDA Approves Epidiolex for Dravet and Lennox-Gastaut Syndromes." 2018.
Federal recognition that a cannabis derivative can meet rigorous approval standards in the United States.

George Washington & Thomas Jefferson
18th Century Writings
Both grew hemp extensively for rope, sails, and oil; their writings underscore hemp's economic and agricultural significance in early America.

Hearst, William Randolph
Hearst Newspapers, 1930s
Launched sensational anti-cannabis propaganda linking the plant to crime and jazz, helping cement early national stigma.

Israel / Canada / Australia National Cannabis Programs
Government Reports (2015-2024)
Registries and prescribing programs showing long-term patient outcomes in epilepsy, pain, MS, and cancer care globally.

Israel Ministry of Health
National Medical Cannabis Program: Annual Report, 2024
Published data on patient outcomes, prescribing trends, and longitudinal monitoring of cannabis therapies.

Jefferson, Thomas
Notes on Hemp Cultivation at Monticello, circa 1774
His agricultural journals document hemp's use for fiber and seed oil in early American farms.

Johns Hopkins University School of Medicine
"Medical Cannabis for PTSD: Outcomes in Real-World Veterans." JAMA Network Open, 2021
Survey-based observational study showing improved sleep, reduced anxiety, and PTSD symptom relief among veteran cannabis users.

Lambert Initiative for Cannabinoid Therapeutics (University of Sydney)
Annual Clinical Review on Cannabinoid Therapy, 2023
An Australian center synthesizing global research, advocating policy reform, and supporting national cannabinoid trials.

Lancet Neurology
"Randomized Controlled Trial of Cannabidiol in Epilepsy." The Lancet Neurology, 2018
A landmark RCT that showed CBD reduced convulsive seizures in treatment-resistant epilepsy populations.

Maccarrone, Mauro et al.
"Endocannabinoid Signaling in the Gut: From Physiology to Therapy." Nature Reviews Gastroenterology & Hepatology, 2020
Explored how gut–brain ECS signaling may be harnessed for GI disorders like IBS and Crohn's.

Mechoulam, Raphael & Y. Gaoni
"Isolation, Structure, and Partial Synthesis of an Active Constituent of Hashish." Journal of the American Chemical Society, 1964
The first chemical isolation and identification of THC, establishing the foundation of cannabis chemistry.

National Academies of Sciences, Engineering, and Medicine
The Health Effects of Cannabis and Cannabinoids: The Current State of Evidence and Recommendations for Research. Washington, D.C.: National Academies Press, 2017
A consensus report reviewing over 10,000 studies; identified substantial evidence for cannabis in chronic pain, chemotherapy nausea, and MS spasticity.

Naftali, Timna et al.
"Cannabis Induces Clinical Remission in Patients with Crohn's Disease." Clinical Gastroenterology and Hepatology, 2013
Found that cannabis use was associated with clinical remission and reduced medication requirement in Crohn's patients.

Neurology Journal
"Smoked Cannabis Reduces Neuropathic Pain in HIV Patients." Neurology, 2007
Demonstrated a one-third reduction in neuropathic pain and paved the way for cannabis analgesic research.

Novack, Gary D
"Cannabinoids and Intraocular Pressure: Review of Mechanisms and Therapeutic Potential." Experimental Eye Research, 2016
Reviewed how cannabinoids modulate aqueous humor and protect retinal ganglion cells in glaucoma models.

Okun, Michael S
"Medical Marijuana and Parkinson's Disease: What Patients Tell Us." Parkinson's Foundation Report, 2022
Surveyed Parkinson's patients; most reported improvements in tremor, stiffness, and quality of life after using cannabis.

Pen Ts'ao Ching (Herbal of the Divine Farmer)
(Attributed to Emperor Shen Nung), 2737 BCE
Ancient Chinese pharmacopoeia referencing ma (cannabis) as medicine for pain, fever, and women's health.

Ramses II Mummy (Egyptian Antiquities Records)
c. 1200 BCE
Detectable cannabis traces were found in tissues and wrappings, emphasizing cannabis's historical ritual and medicinal use in Egypt. While some researchers debate potential contamination during preservation, the findings still demonstrate that cannabis was known and utilized in ritual or medicinal contexts in ancient Egypt.

Reynolds, Sir J. Russell
"On the Therapeutic Uses and Toxic Effects of Cannabis." The Lancet, 1890
As physician to Queen Victoria, Reynolds endorsed cannabis tinctures for menstrual pain, migraines, and insomnia; one of the early Western medical endorsements.

Russo, Ethan B.
Clinical Endocannabinoid Deficiency: Toward Restoring Internal Balance. Neuro Endocrinology Letters, 2004
Reframed how endocannabinoid tone influences conditions like migraines, IBS, fibromyalgia, and introduced the CECD hypothesis.

Sanskrit Origin of "Ananda"
Ancient India
The Sanskrit word Ananda means "bliss," root of Anandamide, the body's natural endocannabinoid.

Scythian Burial Records (Herodotus, The Histories)
Book IV, 440 BCE
Described Scythians using hemp vapor in ceremonial rites; one of the earliest accounts of ritual cannabis inhalation.

Sir J. Russell Reynolds
Physician to Queen Victoria
Included as historical context for cannabis use in 19th-century medical practice (see his 1890 The Lancet article above).

United States Pharmacopeia
"Cannabis Extracts Listed as Official Medicines." Editions 1850–1942
Listed Cannabis sativa in official pharmacopeias for pain, insomnia, and neuralgia prior to federal prohibition.

University of Bristol & Yale University
"CBD Reduces Anxiety in Simulated Public Speaking Tests." Neuropsychopharmacology, 2019
Interventional study showing CBD significantly reduced stress responses in public speaking simulations.

University of Colorado Anschutz Medical Campus
"Medical Cannabis for Migraines: Retrospective Analysis of Clinical Outcomes." Pharmacotherapy, 2019
Found reduced frequency and severity of migraines among patients using medical cannabis.

University of Haifa Clinical Neuroscience Center
"Canneroid Therapy in Alzheimer's and Dementia Care." 2021
Reported improved sleep, agitation, and caregiver burden in dementia patients using cannabinoid treatments.

University of Oxford Neuroscience Group
"Cannabinoids in Multiple Sclerosis: Neuroprotection and Symptom Control." Lancet Neurology, 2015
Found evidence for cannabinoid-induced neuroprotective effects in MS animal models and symptom relief in human cohorts.

University of Tel Aviv Clinical Neuroscience Center
"Cannabinoid Therapy in Alzheimer's and Dementia Care." 2021
Documented real-world outcomes for cannabinoid-assisted treatment of Alzheimer's disease symptoms.

United States Department of Veterans Affairs (VA)
Veterans and Cannabis Use: National Survey Data Summary, 2022
Aggregated national survey data regarding cannabis use, satisfaction, and reported health outcomes among U.S. veterans.

Virginia General Assembly
"Act Requiring Hemp Cultivation." Colonial Records, 1619
Early law mandating hemp cultivation in Virginia; reflects cannabis's agricultural centrality in colonial America.

William C. Woodward, M.D.
Testimony before U.S. Congress opposing the Marihuana Tax Act, 1937
As AMA delegate, he opposed prohibition arguments and warned cannabis had valid medical applications.

World Health Organization (WHO)
Cannabis and Cannabinoids: Critical Review Report. Geneva, 2020
Reaffirmed CBD's safety profile, low abuse potential, and evidence for its therapeutic use in seizures, anxiety, and pain.

World Health Organization (WHO)
Global Status Report on Alcohol and Health. 2023
Used to contextualize substance policy, epidemiology, and public health frameworks within which cannabis policy is debated.

POSTSCRIPT

As this book reached print, the United States witnessed one of the most dramatic policy contradictions in the history of Cannabis and hemp.

On September 28, 2025, President Donald Trump released a video calling on Medicare to cover hemp derived cannabidiol for seniors. He described CBD as a game changer for senior health, citing its ability to restore balance in the body, ease pain, improve sleep, and reduce stress. He urged the federal government to provide coverage for CBD and give millions of older Americans the support they deserve.

For patients, caregivers, physicians, and advocates, it sounded like progress at last.

A rare moment where science, compassion, and federal authority appeared to be moving in the same direction.

Yet only weeks later, in early November 2025, Congress passed a federal amendment that effectively banned most hemp derived cannabinoids nationwide. The law created a new category called "*intoxicating hemp products*," defined so broadly that it captures almost everything produced under the 2018 Farm Bill.

Delta-8, Delta-10, HHC, THCP, converted cannabinoids of any kind, and even full spectrum CBD products that contain natural traces of THC all fall under the new definition. The ban takes effect one year from enactment and will dismantle a multi-billion dollar industry that millions rely on for wellness and relief.

The contradiction is unavoidable to ignore.

In September the nation was told that CBD is medicine. In November the government restricted the very products required to deliver it.

Two policies, released weeks apart, moving in opposite directions. One endorses therapeutic potential. The other eliminates access to it.

This moment captures exactly why this book exists. The science is advancing. Public understanding is growing. But federal policy continues to swing between fear and acceptance, often with no alignment to evidence or reality.

Cannabis: Clearing the Smoke was written to bridge that gap. To trace where the misconceptions came from. To show what modern research actually reveals. And to explain why millions of people turn to this plant not out of rebellion but out of necessity.

The recent federal reversal underscores the urgency of clear and honest education. It is not enough to acknowledge the usefulness of cannabinoids in a speech or a press release. Patients need access. Physicians need clarity. Policymakers need literacy. And the public deserves truth.

Which brings us to where this first book ends and the next begins.

Book Two explores the system that makes all of this possible. The Endocannabinoid System is real. Its potential is vast. And the time for acceptance is now!

www.ingramcontent.com/pod-product-compliance
Lightning Source LLC
Chambersburg PA
CBHW050223270326
41914CB00003BA/546
9798994361016